Practical
MEDICAL
Halachah

FRED ROSNER
MOSHE D. TENDLER

JASON ARONSON INC.
Northvale, New Jersey
Jerusalem

Library of Congress Cataloging-in-Publication Data

Rosner, Fred.
    Practical medical halachah / Fred Rosner and Rav Moshe D. Tendler.
— 3rd rev. ed.
        p.   cm.
    Reprint. Previously published: 1990.
    Includes bibliographical references.
    ISBN 0–7657–9990–1
    1. Medical laws and legislation (Jewish law)   I. Tendler, Moshe
David, 1926–   II. Title.
296.1′8–dc21   97–28714

Manufactured in the United States of America. Jason Aronson Inc. offers books and
cassettes. For information and catalog write to Jason Aronson Inc., 230 Livingston
Street, Northvale, NJ 07647.

In Memoriam

כשמת רבי אליעזר רבי עקיבא . . .
פתח עליו בשורה ואמר הרבה מעות יש לי
ואין לי שולחני להרצותן

(Babylonian Talmud, *Sanhedrin* 78a)

When R. Eliezer died, R. Akiva eulogized him thus:
I have many coins
but there is no one to exchange them.

Rashi explains this simile:
I have so many questions to ask,
but with the passing of our rabbi,
there is no one to answer them.

Contents

CIRCUMCISION

DEATH AND DYING

HAZARDOUS THERAPY AND HUMAN EXPERIMENTATION

MENTAL HEALTH

MISCELLANEOUS QUESTIONS

PREFACE

Cellular maturation is a complex biological process. In relation to man and his institutions, maturation is an equally complex social process whose stages are apparent to the astute observer.

This compilation of *Halachah Bulletins* is evidence of the maturation of the Rephael Society, the Health Care Section of the Association of Orthodox Jewish Scientists. More significantly, it is also a sign of the maturation taking place in the Torah community of the United States. In these bulletins the central concerns, interests, and commitments of the medical and dental professionals of our community are evident. Their calls for assistance in dealing with ethical and moral issues are met in a clear, definitive fashion with halachic response that are intended to be helpful in a direct, practical way. This dynamic interaction of science and *halachah* demonstrates that Torah-directed life is not an abstract concept but a viable alternative that is professionally acceptable, socially feasible, and personally desirable.

The terminology, subject matter, and concise style of these bulletins clearly identify them as intended solely for a professional readership. They are not intended for the general layman interested in *halachah* whose medical background is not adequate to prevent misinterpretations and misunderstanding. They were issued as "first aid" measures for our physicians and dentists in need of guidance on the critical halachic issues they confront daily.

The halachic decisions as published were arrived at by traditional *she'elah-teshuvah* techniques. Because of the far-reaching significance of many of these halachic decisions, they were submitted to HaGaon Rav Moshe Feinstein of blessed memory for review. The language and analyses, however, are those of the authors, who bear sole responsibility for the accuracy of the contents.

The first edition of this booklet on practical medical *halachah* was published in 1974 and the second edition in 1980. Much has happened in medical ethics, and the need for the Jewish view to be heard has increased. The demand by members of the Rephael Society for previous *Halachah Bulletins* and for additional medical halachic material has prompted us to prepare this enlarged and revised edition. The organization of the material has been somewhat modified from the earlier edition to assist in the smooth flow of subjects and concepts. The additional *Halachah Bulletins* of the past several years have been incorporated into the booklet, and an essay on dental emergencies on the Sabbath has been included. Furthermore, this booklet addresses the importance of and controversy about the definition of death in *halachah* in a full-length article entitled "Physiologic Decapitation as a Definition of Death in Judaism." The related issue of "brain absent" anencephalics and their possible use as organ donors is also discussed in some detail.

We hope that physicians, dentists, and other members of the health care professions will derive benefit from this booklet, clearly recognizing that its intent is not to provide annotated and detailed presentations of medical halachic material. Rather, our goal is to offer a general framework for the practicing health professional that may serve as a starting point for more in-depth study and investigation of important issues in Jewish medical ethics.

Fred Rosner, M.D.
Rav Moshe D. Tendler, Ph.D.

FOREWORD

The great medical advances that have occurred over the past few decades boggle the minds of even the most progressive scientists. Strides in the fields of prolongation of life, genetic engineering, neonatology, and in-utero diagnostics and therapy, to name a few, have created new dilemmas for the orthodox Jewish health care professional. In addition, other pressures have been brought to bear by the nonmedical aspects of health care today. Utilization review, quality assurance, malpractice, and other concepts are now influencing the way health care is delivered. Cost containment by government and profit motives of hospitals have altered the basic environment in the delivery of health care. Increasing regulations, increasing frustrations, decreasing satisfactions, and the perceived decreasing sanctity of life, vis-à-vis the "rights" of the individual and society, have detracted from the aura of health care delivery.

And yet, the orthodox Jewish professional knows the great value placed on the saving of a single human life. Indeed, the infinite value of a moment of life transcends all the petty bureaucracy associated with its preservation. Questions posed by *frum* health care deliverers revolve not around the mundane, but rather around scientific knowledge as it interfaces with the sanctity of the Torah. The third edition of *Practical Medical Halachah* represents the ongoing evolution of *she'elot-teshuvot* posed by the orthodox medical community and answered by the halachic giant of our generation, HaGaon Rav Moshe Feinstein zt"l. Dr. Fred Rosner and Rabbi Dr. Moshe Tendler continue to gather praise as they review, edit, and embellish the previous editions of *Practical Medical Halachah*. May they continue to provide insight and answers to the ever-growing need for Torah-true direction in the difficult path on which health care delivery finds itself.

HaGaon Rav Moshe Feinstein zt"l served not only as the posek for the Rephael Society but for all Israel as well. His rulings were accepted by all, his decisions were based on solid halachic ground, and his p'sak was guided by the compassion befitting the *Gadol Hador*, the leader of the generation, that he was. His teaching will live on in all subsequent editions through the responsa of his son-in-law, Rav Dr. Moshe Tendler, his *talmid muvhak* (devoted pupil) for more than thirty years. Rav Feinstein's passing has created a vacuum in halachic decision-making from which we struggle to recover. It is only fitting that this volume be dedicated to his memory.

In conclusion, the orthodox professional should be aware that this compendium serves as a guide only. All questions pertaining to actual cases should be directed to a *rav* competent in medical/halachic fundamentals for adjudication. The ethical basis of this work will guide orthodox health care professionals as they face the ever-increasing perplexities of the medical/halachic interface as we approach the twenty-first century.

May we all be privileged to speedily see the time of the coming of the Messiah and the resolution of the ethical dilemmas that face the orthodox health care community in its attempts to practice its vocation in the ways of the Torah.

Allen J. Bennett, M.D.
President,
Association of Orthodox
Jewish Scientists

THE PHYSICIANS'

LICENSE TO HEAL

Subject: *Halachic definition of a physician.*

Question: Is a third- or fourth-year medical student (clinical clerk) considered a full-fledged physician for halachic purposes? What is the role of a medical student? What is the halachic definition of a physician? What is the role of the nurse?

Answer: A medical student has the same halachic coverage as a house staff physician or attending physician.

Comment: Although the student has no legal responsibility for patient care, and although he may not have adequate knowledge to exercise mature medical judgment, his aid is often necessary and nearly always beneficial. Time is saved by the senior physician because additional hands are available. The *halachah* does not distinguish between medical student, clinical clerk, intern, resident, and attending physician, or even layman, insofar as all contribute to the total patient care. The obligation to aid a dangerously ill patient falls not only on the graduate physician but on anyone able to and asked to render assistance. Included in this obligation are first- and second-year medical students and certainly third- and fourth-year students who possess considerable medical knowledge and are essential members of the diagnostic and therapeutic team.

The industrious and aggressive medical student may have access to information that may be extremely recent and not clearly known to the senior physicians in attendance. The student may be able to devote many hours to an individual patient, thus making him the patient's "primary" doctor. The student's long and detailed history and physical examination may reveal facts and physical findings that might otherwise have been missed. The additional period of questioning may allow the patient to reflect and remember more important information not elicited by the other examiners. By performing many other required tasks, the student enables the physician to render better care to the patient. For these reasons, a medical student has the same halachic coverage as the graduate physician, including laws pertaining to the Sabbath and *Yom Tov*.

Similarly, a nurse administering therapy or supportive care under a physician's direction is considered a member of the health care team with respect to halachic license to treat patients on the Sabbath.

Source: Shulchan Aruch, Orach Chayim 328:10.

Subject: *Kohen (priest) studying medicine.*

Question: May a *kohen* study medicine? What restrictions or permissive rulings, if any, are there regarding this question?

Answer: A *kohen* in the United States is *prohibited* from attending medical school.

Comment: Because of the requirement in United States medical schools that students take anatomy and pathology courses, there is no way that a *kohen* can attend medical school without violating *halachah*. Even if the assumption is made that most if not all cadavers are non-Jewish, ritual defilement of a *kohen* still occurs upon contact with any dead body, although a non-Jewish cadaver does not ritually defile those people present in the same room who are not in physical contact with the deceased.

Although the exemption of *pikuach nefesh* (danger to life) sets aside all the commandments in the Torah (except the cardinal three), permissive rulings based on this principle apply *only* to physicians already in practice who are *kohanim*. The consideration of potential *pikuach nefesh* does *not*, however, sanction a *kohen* to begin medical school where the above-cited halachic problem cannot be overcome.

The rumored permissive ruling of the late Chief Rabbi Isaac Herzog, based on the promise to settle in Israel and contribute to the medical needs of the developing state, has never been confirmed in writing and, therefore, cannot be given any credence.

Subject: *Kohen (priest) studying dentistry.*

Question: May a *kohen* become a dentist? What restrictions or permissive rulings, if any, are there regarding this question?

Answer: Under the usual academic conditions, a *kohen* is *not* permitted to study dentistry.

Comment: In the previous answer, we pointed out that, because of the requirement in United States medical schools that students take anatomy and pathology courses, there is no way that a *kohen* can attend medical school without violating *halachah*. Even if the assumption is made that most, if not all, cadavers are non-Jewish, ritual defilement of a *kohen* still occurs upon contact (*maga*) or by carrying (*massa*) *any* dead body. The halachic distinction between Jew and Gentile concerns ritual defilement on being present in the same room with a cadaver (*tumat ohel*).

The same objections concerning medical school apply to dental school. The latter curriculum also includes anatomical dissection, which is forbidden to a *kohen* irrespective of whether the cadaver is Jewish or non-Jewish. If, however, the dental student can avoid actual dissection and attend only as an observer and if his early dentistry training does not include a human skull with its dentition, then there is little halachic objection to a *kohen* studying dentistry. This restricted permissibility rests upon the fact that in the present era we follow the lenient halachic ruling that a non-Jewish corpse does not convey ritual defilement to people in the same room who have no direct contact with it. Unlike the physician, the dentist is not usually involved with dying patients, death certificates, the mortuary, etc., which pose seemingly insoluble problems to a physician who is a *kohen*.

Source: Karo's *Shulchan Aruch, Yoreh Deah* 369, 371, and 372:2 and the commentary *Dagul Mervavah* on the last reference.

Subject: *Nonphysician kohen (priest) working in a hospital.*

Question: Is a *kohen* permitted to accept employment in a hospital (since contact with a dead body or even the presence in the same room of a Jewish deceased ritually defiles the *kohen*)?

Answer and Comment: If a *kohen* is offered a position in a hospital and, if a patient dies there, the *kohen* is unable to leave but must tend to the other patients even in other rooms, he is not allowed to accept that position. Even if we accept the reasoning (*Sifsei Cohen, Yoreh Deah* 372:2) that ritual defilement of a dead body transmitted to another house (or room) is only a rabbinic (and not biblical) concept, one still cannot permit a *kohen* to accept such a position in a hospital even if he thereby incurs considerable financial loss, because even a rabbinic prohibition cannot be set aside because of monetary considerations.

Furthermore, not all rabbis agree with the Sifsei Cohen and many consider ritual defilement of a *kohen* by a corpse in an adjoining room or house to be biblical in nature. Therefore it is prohibited for a *kohen* to accept a position in a hospital if it is absolutely certain that he must remain if there is a Jewish deceased there. However, if he can stipulate that he can leave if a Jewish corpse is present in the hospital, and if there are not many Jewish patients in that hospital so that on most days there is no Jewish corpse there, then it is permissible to work in that hospital. One considers the fact that most patients recover and it is no different from a *kohen* entering a large house or a place where there is a large gathering of people. One is not concerned lest one of the assemblage die and the *kohen* become defiled; so too, for the *kohen* working in a hospital where there is not an overwhelming majority of Jewish patients. However, if the *kohen* knows that there is a Jewish patient on the verge of death, the *kohen* should leave the hospital.

Reference: Feinstein, M. *Iggrot Moshe, Yoreh Deah,* Responsum 248, New York, 1959, p. 509.

Subject: *Genetic counselling as a profession for an orthodox Jew.*

Question: Are there restrictions that might preclude an orthodox Jewish man or woman from pursuing a career in genetic counselling?

Answer and Comment: There are no halachic restrictions that preclude one from studying and practicing genetic counselling. Genetic counselling is becoming an increasingly complex and specialized discipline requiring an understanding by the physician or counsellor of genes as etiologic agents of disease, of the effect of drugs, of the effect of maternal or paternal age, of the effect of radiation and viruses such as rubella and influenza, of specialized laboratory procedures available for the diagnosis of carrier states, of chromosomal analysis and amniocentesis, of sophisticated techniques now available for prenatal testing including the direct examination of the unborn fetus's blood, and of possible treatment available for genetic disorders.

Genetic counselling includes the provision of information concerning diagnosis, prognosis, and statistical probability of recurrence. The delivery of that information is central to the task of the counsellor. The manner of delivery and the content of the information and the style with which it is presented are all of paramount importance. Psychological, psychiatric, and religious considerations must be taken into account. Counselling not only involves semantics but touches on values and beliefs. Counselling must be personal. It cannot be directive, but must be fully informative. Decisions of young couples are greatly influenced and modified by the persuasive efforts of the physician and the authoritarian statements of the rabbi or religious counsellor. The birth of a child with a serious congenital deformity, or mental deficiency, or a lethal metabolic error such as Tay-Sachs disease is a terrible shock to any parent. The personal decisions involved are very difficult: whether to marry; whether to have children; whether to have a further child; whether to adopt a child. For Jewish patients, not only must medical, genetic, and psychological factors be considered in any given case, but the religious attitude of Judaism toward such matters as abortion, contraception, amniocentesis, genetic screening, and procreation, to name but a few, must be taken into account.

The orthodox Jewish counsellor should emphasize the sanctity of life and other basic principles of Judaism and its religious orientation. If the final decision made by the patient(s) is contrary to Jewish law, the counsellor bears no responsibility. If the counsellor is unable to convince the patient or client of the Torah view, at least the counsellor tried. If possible and when appropriate, rabbinic consultation and advice should be sought concomitantly with the medical-genetic counselling.

Subject: *A physician or dentist treating his own family, including his parents.*

Question: Is a physician or dentist permitted to diagnose and treat illness in close members of his own family? Does the ruling apply equally to parent, sibling, spouse, child, aunt, uncle, cousin, nephew, niece, etc.? Is a physician permitted to perform a complete physical examination on his close relative? May a physician or dentist draw blood from, or perform surgery on, or administer medication to his parents?

Answer: A physician or dentist should *not* draw blood, give injections, or perform surgery (even *minor*) on his *parents*, but may do so for *all* other relatives. If a life-threatening medical emergency arises, a physician may treat his parents, if no equally competent physician is available.

Comment: No greater honor can a Jewish physician bestow upon his father and mother than diagnosing and treating their physical ailments, particularly if the parent has more confidence in the child than in other physicians. Thus, all diagnostic and therapeutic procedures, including history-taking, physical examination, and prescribing treatment, are allowed in the fulfillment of *Honor thy father and mother.* Because of emotional involvement with family, the advice and cooperation of a colleague is recommended.

There is, however, a biblical prohibition against inflicting a wound upon one's parent, and therefore any diagnostic procedure that involves drawing blood, giving injections, lancing boils, or other minor or major surgery, all of which are considered to constitute a "wound," should *not* be performed by a physician or dentist, unless no equally competent physician or dentist is available.

No such restriction exists for all other relatives, including siblings, cousins, aunts, uncles, nephews, children, and spouses! However, when one's wife is a *niddah*, it is forbidden to examine her unless there is a life-threatening emergency.

Source: *Shulchan Aruch, Yoreh Deah, Ramah 241:2.*

PROCREATION

AND SEXUALITY

Subject: *Gynecological diagnostic procedures.*

Question: Does a pelvic examination or Pap smear or endometrial biopsy or I.U.D. insertion with or without resultant bleeding render a woman *niddah*?

Answer: Bleeding following a pelvic examination does not necessarily render a woman *niddah*.

Comment:
a) *Pelvic examinations.*

When a gynecologist finds it necessary to perform a pelvic examination on a Jewish woman patient, any bleeding that may ensue from the physical irritation of the examination is not considered to be menstrual blood necessitating abstinence. However, if for any reason it is necessary to pass an instrument past the cervical os into the cervical canal, the Jewish patient must be so advised. If the instrument is 0.7 inches in diameter (1.75 cm) or more, the patient must consider herself to be a *niddah* even if *no* bleeding ensues. Bleeding from cervical erosions or the cauterization used to treat these erosions is *not* considered *niddah* blood. If feasible, pelvic examination should be done within twenty-four hours prior to onset of menses. It is necessary for the patient to consult with her rabbi to determine the regulations that she must observe following pelvic examinations.

b) *Pap smear.*

In the usual procedure no instrument penetrates the cervical os. The cotton swab and wooden applicator stick are of such dimensions as to present no halachic concerns.

c) *Endometrial biopsy.*

Although the uterine cavity is entered in endometrial biopsy, the instrument is usually less than 6 mm in diameter and therefore does not cause *psichat hakever* (cervical dilation). Therefore, the patient is not considered a *niddah*.

d) *I.U.D. insertion.*

The cervix is usually dilated to permit insertion of an intrauterine contraceptive device. Even if no bleeding occurs, the patient becomes a *niddah*.

e) *Hysterogram.*

The radioopaque dye used to infuse the uterus is administered via a cannula only a few millimeters in diameter. Thus there is no *psichat hakever* and the *niddah* state is not induced.

Subject: *Contraception.*

Question: Under what circumstances, if any, may contraceptive methods be employed? Which methods are most preferable in Jewish law?

Answer: Contraceptive methods may be used only for specific medical or psychiatric indications.

Comment: Contraceptive devices cannot be used except for specific medical indications such as rheumatic heart disease, severe renal disease, and similar situations, where pregnancy would constitute a serious threat to the health of the mother. Jewish law requires that the marital act be as normal as possible. When medical indications, which include psychological factors, necessitate the use of a contraceptive technique, Jewish law grades methods of contraceptive techniques from least to most objectionable in the following order: oral contraceptives, chemical spermicidals, diaphragms and cervical caps to be used by the wife, condoms, and coitus interruptus. The most objectionable method, and one that is least often permitted under Jewish law, is the use by the male of the condom or withdrawal.

An intrauterine contraceptive device (I.U.D.) cannot be sanctioned by Jewish law. Their propensity for inducing intermenstrual spotting is a significant deterrent to their use. In addition the risk of uterine perforations and pelvic infections violates the law of *ushmartem* that instructs us to avoid all risks to health.

Subject: *Contraceptive advice to unmarried girls.*

Question: Does *halachah* permit an orthodox Jewish physician to give contraceptive advice to and to prescribe contraceptive devices for unmarried girls?

Answer: Except under very exceptional circumstances, Judaism considers it immoral for the physician to give contraceptive advice to an unmarried girl.

Comment: The doctor must use judicious moral judgment in this sensitive area of human relations. Judaism deems it immoral to give contraceptive counsel to unmarried persons when such advice may serve to remove a significant barrier to immoral conduct. When confronted with the mentally retarded patient or with people in whom self-discipline is lacking as determined by previous conduct, consultation with a religious guide should be undertaken to decide the proper course of action.

Subject: *Sperm procurement and analysis.*

Question: Is sperm analysis permissible in Jewish law? Under what circumstances? How should one obtain the sperm?

Answer: Sperm analysis is allowed when medically indicated, provided the sperm is obtained as described below.

Comment: During the medical workup of a sterility problem, it is occasionally necessary to test the semen of the husband for quantity and quality of sperm. The least objectionable method is the procurement of sperm by coitus interruptus, or if this is unsatisfactory for any reason, a condom may be applied on the male membrum prior to coitus. These two procedures involve the natural sex act and are, therefore, most acceptable to Jewish law. Masturbation to obtain sperm is strongly condemned, based upon the following talmudic passage: ". . . Rabbi Eleazer stated: Who are referred to in the scriptural text *Your hands are full of blood* (Isaiah 1:15)? Those that commit masturbation with their hands. It was taught at the School of Rabbi Ishmael: *Thou shalt not commit adultery* (Exod. 20:13) implies that thou shalt not practice masturbation either with hand or with foot. . . ." The use of a mechanical vibrator applied to the *anal* area to induce erection and ejaculation to procure semen for examination can also be approved, if necessary.

To have sexual intercourse in the physician's office so that the physician can retrieve the sperm from the vagina of the woman is considered licentious and improper. When it is necessary to evaluate sperm survival in the vaginal tract, a nearby hotel room must be obtained to enable the wife to present herself shortly after coitus for such testing. Of course, the laws of *niddah* must be observed even under these medical conditions.

Source: *Shulchan Aruch, Even Ha'ezer* 23:1–3

Subject: *Artificial insemination.*

Question: Is artificial insemination ever allowed in Jewish law Under what circumstances? Is the ruling different depending upon whether donor sperm or the husband's sperm is used?

Answer: Under most circumstances, artificial insemination using donor sperm is not permitted. Semen from the husband may be used to impregnate his wife if there is adequate medical reason to use a high uterine insemination instead of normal cohabitation.

Comment: Artificial insemination using the semen of a donor other than the husband (A.I.D.) is considered by most rabbinic opinion to be strictly prohibited for a variety of reasons, including the possibility of incest, confused genealogy, and the problems of inheritance. However, without a sexual act involved, the woman is not guilty of adultery, and is not prohibited to cohabit with her husband. The child born from A.I.D. does not carry any stigma of illegitimacy. The use of semen from the husband is permissible if no other method is possible for the wife to become pregnant. If the insemination must be performed during the wife's period of ritual impurity, stored semen may be used but consultation with a rabbinic authority is required.

Since many important legal and moral considerations that cannot be enunciated in the presentation of these general principles may weigh heavily upon the verdict in any given situation, it is essential that each individual case be submitted to rabbinic judgment that, in turn, will be based upon expert medical opinion, both physiological and psychological.

Subject: *Induction of labor.*

Question: Is there a halachic objection to inducing labor by means of oxytocin or prostaglandins?

Answer and Comment: If induction of labor is undertaken for clinical indications of major obstetric complications, that is to say the welfare of the mother or child, it is certainly permissible. Such situations might include severe pre-eclampsia, diabetes mellitus, bleeding, overdue babies, blood group incompatibility, or the like, according to the judgment of the obstetrician.

Any medical or surgical procedure that is carried out for any purpose other than the benefit of the patient constitutes assault and battery. Hence, induction of labor undertaken for the social convenience of the mother and/or obstetrician is contrary to *halachah*. *Halachah* clearly forbids any procedure that carries additional risk to mother or child. Induction of labor for social convenience may well involve increased risk to the baby or mother and, hence, would constitute an unethical procedure in the eyes of Jewish law.

The following is a quotation from an editorial in the prestigious medical journal *Lancet* (Nov. 16, 1974, pp. 1183–4):

> . . . induction on the grounds of social convenience is a pernicious practice which has no place in modern obstetrics. The mother's holiday, the calls of the obstetrician's private practice, must not influence, for the sake of even a few days, an event which for the child may affect the outcome of its entire life. Social convenience must be dismissed. Medical convenience—daylight delivery—is a more difficult problem; the argument goes as follows: The chances of the occurrence of a major life-threatening emergency are greater at delivery than at any other time of life. If one could choose the time of one's road accident, coronary thrombosis, or gastrointestinal haemorrhage, it would be at 10 A.M. on a Tuesday in October. No-one is asleep, on holiday, or a dozen miles away. Obstetric complications offer, in principle, a similar choice: a median delivery-time of 5 P.M. on a weekday could be achieved for at least half the population. Should this be the aim? The question cannot be easily answered at present.
>
> Indeed, there is even some evidence that foetal complications, as judged by the need for incubation or oxygen administration, may be relatively more common during daylight hours.
>
> Further observations and information are essential if an objective

answer is to be found to the question whether or not induction of labor for medical convenience is sound clinical practice or meddlesome midwifery. If it really is more dangerous to be born at night, either we should make daylight delivery the norm to aim for, or we should ensure that the same facilities are available by night as during the day.

Halachah requires the latter course; namely to have all the necessary facilities available at night as well. The possibility of better response to an emergency situation during daylight hours is no justification for introducing a procedure (i.e., induction of labor) that, in itself, may be less than "good medical practice." Induction of labor should be reserved only for those clinical conditions that demand early termination of pregnancy so as to benefit mother or child.

Once labor has begun, the judgment of the obstetrician determines the need for oxytocin for the benefit of mother and/or child.

Subject: *Assistance of husband during natural childbirth.*

Question: Is a husband permitted to assist during natural childbirth (as in the Lamaze method)? When is the wife considered a *niddah* or a *yoledet* (parturient woman)? Is the husband's role during natural childbirth an exemption from the usual laws of *niddah* because of his contribution to his wife's physical and psychological welfare?

Answer: Within certain guidelines (see below) the husband is permitted to be present during natural childbirth and to provide solace and comfort to his wife.

Comment: The wife is considered a *niddah* or a *yoledet* immediately upon the appearance of any blood, the "bloody show," mucus plug tinged with blood, or any active bleeding from the cervical canal. She is also considered a *yoledet* if there is no bleeding at all but labor has progressed to a point of:

a) contractions of such frequency and/or severity to make it very difficult to walk without assistance.

b) the nurse or physicians report that the cervix is fully dilated. Under the above conditions, the *niddah* state is established with all its halachic restrictions.

Prior to that time (i.e., during labor), if no blood has appeared, the woman is not a *niddah* and may even have physical contact with her husband. When she becomes a *niddah*, however, as defined above, no further physical contact is permitted.

Although the hospital environment, the presence of the medical team members, and the preoccupation of both husband and wife with the birth process minimize the halachic concern, lest physical contact lead to forbidden intimacies, it is *not permitted* for the husband to "wipe her face, rub her back, or support her during contraction." Indeed, proper preparations for natural childbirth should include the husband's supportive role—but without physical contact. His presence, encouragement, and reassurances are the sum total of his contributions. Any physical ministrations can better be performed by hospital personnel.

In the delivery room itself, the husband should not view the act of birth of the child but should stand near the head of the table and offer encouragement and reassurance to his wife. He should not even view the birth process through the mirrors present in most delivery rooms.

Subject: *Therapeutic abortion and assisting at an abortion.*

Question: Is therapeutic abortion permitted in Jewish law? If yes, under what circumstances? Is abortion on demand allowed?

May a nurse or anesthesiologist or some other person assist in the performance of an abortion? If they may, under what circumstances? What of a non-Jewish woman who requests an abortion?

Answer: Jewish law sanctions abortions only where a serious hazard to the mother's physical or mental health exists.

Comment: Abortion on demand is prohibited by Jewish law. Jewish law sanctions abortion only when continuation of pregnancy constitutes a grave hazard to the mother. Such hazards include psychiatric disturbances that may be caused or aggravated by the continued pregnancy, if these disturbances are genuinely feared to lead to risk to life. For example, if a woman seriously threatens suicide, and if competent psychiatric opinion agrees with the possibility of danger to the woman's life, then an abortion not only may but must be carried out to save the mother, since her life takes precedence over that of her unborn child. A serious medical threat to the mother's life such as advanced rheumatic heart disease or serious kidney malfunctioning also constitutes an indication for abortion permitted by Jewish law.

The fear that a child might be born physically malformed or mentally deficient, such as following exposure to rubella early in pregnancy or ingestion of thalidomide, or evidence of malformation on ultrasound examination, does not in itself justify recourse to abortion. Both before and after birth, an abnormal child (physically or mentally) enjoys the same title to life as a healthy child. This consideration is quite apart from the chance that an abortion might eliminate a perfectly normal child. The sole indication for terminating a pregnancy in Jewish law is a threat to the mother's physical or mental health that endangers her life.

Request for abortion by Jewess or non-Jewess in no way removes the prohibitions involved. Neither the obstetrician-gynecologist or anesthesiologist or nurse nor any other person may perform or assist in any manner in such abortions unless the life-saving considerations for the mother warrant a halachically approved abortion. The prohibition of performing abortion is a Noachian law and is therefore equally applicable to non-Jewish physicians, based on the scriptural verse *whoso sheddeth the blood of man in man, his blood shall be shed* (Genesis 9:6).

Since many important Jewish legal and moral considerations that cannot be spelled out in the presentation of general principles may weigh upon the verdict in any given case, it is essential to submit every case to rabbinic judgment.

Subject: *Pregnancy reduction.*

Question: Does Judaism sanction pregnancy reduction in multiple gestation under any circumstances? Is the abortion of one or more fetuses with a serious genetic or other disease or defect permissible to allow the other normal fetus or fetuses to be born healthy? Is the selective reduction to two or three normal fetuses from quadruplets, quintuplets, sextuplets, or more permissible to allow the others to be born healthy? Since the chances of salvaging healthy infants in women with five or more fetuses are extremely poor, can all the fetuses be aborted? Is it permissible to selectively abort a fetus who is endangering the life of the mother and perhaps the lives or health of the other fetuses as well?

Answer and Comment: The recent advent of in vitro fertilization and the induction of ovulation by hormones has resulted in the not infrequent occurrence of multiple gestations in which pregnant women may be carrying up to seven or eight fetuses at one time. The incidence of maternal morbidity and mortality is much higher in multiple pregnancy than in single pregnancy. Pregnancy reduction, that is, the intrauterine destruction of some of the fetuses so that the others might live is an option frequently suggested to the prospective parents. This option is offered to reduce the high risk of maternal complications as well as to reduce the high fetal morbidity and mortality associated with multiple pregnancy.

Judaism does not sanction termination of pregnancy for the sake of the fetus. Therefore, grounds for permissibility of pregnancy reduction must rest on the consideration that continuation of a multiple pregnancy constitutes a significant hazard to the health and/or life of the mother. Another area of leniency in Jewish law might be the first forty days after conception during which time considerable rabbinic opinion permits abortion even in the absence of a clear threat to the mother's health or life because prior to forty days the small embryo is not considered to have a firm claim on life. This is especially so when each embryo is endangered by the presence of the others.

In multiple pregnancies, medical technology using ultrasonic guidance is sufficiently sophisticated today to allow the gynecologist to successfully perform pregnancy reduction prior to forty days after conception. Therefore, since most rabbis permit termination of pregnancy during this period even without a strong maternal medical indication, it seems likely that they will be lenient and allow the destruction of some embryos before forty days in order to allow the others to mature and be born healthy.

Subject: *Research on aborted fetuses.*

Question: Is it permissible to perform medical research on a spontaneously or therapeutically aborted fetus? If the fetus is alive? If the fetus is dead?

Answer: No, if the fetus is alive; yes, if the fetus is dead.

Comment: If the fetus is alive, although not viable because of prematurity or malformation, it is considered to be a living person in all respects. Any research activities that might shorten the life of this fetus are absolutely prohibited.

If the abortus is dead as defined by halachic criteria (absence of spontaneous respiration and absence of cardiovascular pulsations), then there does not exist any biblical requirement for burial. However, it is desirable to secure the fetus for burial, in order to preserve the dignity of man "created in God's image" and the sanctity of the dead. Since there is no absolute halachic requirement for burial, for cogent and critical medical research a dead fetus may be used without halachic objection.

Subject: *Sterilization of humans (vasectomy, orchiectomy, tubal ligation, hysterectomy, oophorectomy).*

Question: Is sterilization of a man or a woman permissible in Jewish law? Is ligation of the vas deferens during prostatectomy permissible? Is oophorectomy or orchiectomy for malignant disease allowed?

Answer: Only in cases of absolute medical need is a sterilizing procedure (ligation of Fallopian tubes or vas deferens) or ablative sterilization by surgical or medical means (radiation or drugs) permissible. Only in cases of absolute medical need is vasectomy or orchiectomy permitted. Sterilization of women is permitted in Jewish law when medically imperative.

Comment: Surgical or physical impairment of the reproductive organs of any living creature violates Jewish law, except in cases of urgent medical necessity. In the case of males, upon whom the biblical commandment of *be fruitful and multiply* rests, only a risk to life (e.g., cancer), can justify such procedures; hence, unless medically demanded, the ligation of the vas deferens during prostatectomy should be avoided. The prohibition against impairing the male reproductive organs and functions is unrelated to man's fertility. It applies even to a man known to have become sterile or impotent, whether by reason of age or of anatomic or physiologic aberration that has occurred after birth. If he was born sterile, the above prohibition may not apply.

Vasectomy as a "population control" technique is not condoned in *halachah*. It is forbidden to assist at such surgery in any way on man or animal.

The halachic evaluation of new experimental techniques, such as gold valves and silicon plugs, and the impact of "reversible vasectomies" by virtue of new surgical procedures is not yet complete. The initial opinion is that they cannot be condoned, but more study is needed. It is prohibited for a male to ingest a sterilizing potion (hormonal or cytotoxic), and the physician may not prescribe such a medication for men.

Although the biblical commandment to *be fruitful and multiply* rests primarily on the male, the sterilization of females is permitted only when medically imperative. Rabbinic opinion, as well as the consent of the husband, should always be secured prior to considering ligation of the Fallopian tubes or other surgical procedure leading to sterility. Contraceptive techniques such as diaphragm with spermicidals should be evaluated before the decision to intervene surgically is made. Hysterectomy and/or oophorectomy for cancer therapy is obviously permitted.

Subject: *Sterilization of animals.*

Question: Is sterilization of animals permissible in Jewish law?

Answer and Comment: It is prohibited in Jewish law to surgically or physically impair the reproductive organs of any living creature, male or female; human, animal, fowl, or beast, except in cases of urgent medical necessity. This law makes it difficult for an observant Jew to practice as a veterinarian, since the castration and spaying of animals is a major part of urban veterinary practice. It is also forbidden to instruct a non-Jew to castrate or spay one's animal.

Source: *Shulchan Aruch, Even Ha'ezer 5:11–14.*

Subject: *Medical management of infants with ambiguous genitalia.*

Question: How does one halachically approach a child with ambiguous genitalia? Do psychological considerations play a role in the decision to "make" the child into a boy or a girl?

Answer and Comment: The sex determination of an infant or child with ambiguous genitalia must be based on cytological and genetic (i.e., medical) evidence, *not* on psychological considerations. The presence of testes is to be considered an absolute sign of maleness.

A genetically male infant must *not* be surgically modified to permit rearing him as a female. His inability to function as the male partner in marital relations is not adequate justification for such a sex change. In true hermaphroditism, or when no clearly differentiated gonad is evident, the decision as to the sex identity of the child must be arrived at by careful consultation with competent medical and rabbinic authorities.

Sources: Rashi in *Chagigah* 4a, s.v. *keshebeitzim mibachutz.*

CIRCUMCISION

Subject: *Mogen (Bronstein) circumcision clamp.*

Question: Is it permissible to use the *Mogen* clamp for circumcision? Is a circumcision performed with the *Mogen* clamp valid in Jewish law? Is there a prohibition against the use of the *Mogen* clamp?

Answer: The *Mogen* clamp should *not* be used to perform ritual circumcision.

Comment: There are two major objections to the use of the *Mogen* clamp for circumcision.

1. If the clamp is left on for an extended period of time (more than a few minutes), complete hemostasis will result so that no free blood flow occurs. This would invalidate the circumcision.
2. The use of clamps (*Mogen*, Gomco, Cantor, etc.) might lead to circumcision becoming a surgical rather than a ritual procedure, performed by nonorthodox physicians, clergymen, or laymen rather than by an orthodox Jew.

For the above reasons, the *Mogen* clamp should *not* be used. Circumcisions performed in the past with the *Mogen* clamp in which the clamp was applied for only a very brief time (less than a minute), so that blood flow (*hatafat dam*) was not impeded, are perfectly valid in Jewish law, and no question should be raised as to the *kashrut* thereof.

It is recommended that a simple shield or butterfly be used as a guard for ritual circumcision.

Subject: *Circumcision of a hemophiliac.*

Question: Is it permissible for a *mohel* to perform a circumcision on a baby who is known to have hemophilia, or whose brothers or maternal uncles or cousins are know to have hemophilia? Can such a procedure be performed halachically in today's era of fresh frozen plasma, cryoprecipitate, and other factor VIII concentrates, where the danger of bleeding is markedly reduced?

Answer: A hemophilic child may *not* be circumcised until after the perinatal period and only if a competent hematologist is present and confident that the child is adequately protected by the blood fractions he administers.

Comment: The Talmud (Yebamot 64b), as well as the Codes of Jewish law including Maimonides and Karo, rule that the third child of a woman whose two earlier sons had died as a result of circumcision may not be circumcised.

In this day of hematological sophistication where antihemophilic globulin (factor VIII) assays can establish the diagnosis of hemophilia at or shortly after birth, one is not permitted to circumcise any child so diagnosed, even if he didn't have older siblings who exsanguinated after this operation. A positive diagnosis established by the finding of low or absent antihemophilic globulin levels in the plasma of a newborn infant is equivalent in Jewish law to a history of two siblings having died after circumcision. A woman whose brothers bled to death after circumcision cannot have her son circumcised until the coagulation studies on her son are shown to be normal.

With the advent of fresh frozen plasma and cryoprecipitate for the treatment of hemophilia, one might consider elective circumcision. However, in spite of these therapeutic aids, the risks of bleeding after the operation are still substantially greater in a hemophilic child than a normal infant. Thus, in Jewish law, one must postpone this operation and abide by the rule enunciated by Maimonides (*Hilchot Milah* 1:18): ". . . one may circumcise only a child that is totally free of disease, because danger to life overrides every other consideration. *It is possible to circumcise later* than the proper time when the perinatal period is over and the danger of prolonged bleeding of the otherwise healthy child is no longer viewed as potentially life-threatening, but it is impossible to restore a single (departed) soul of Israel forever."

A full discussion of hemophilia in the Talmud and rabbinic writings appeared in the *Annals of Internal Medicine*, Volume 70, No. 4, pages 833–837, April, 1969.

Subject: *Metzitzah (sucking) in ritual circumcision.*

Question: Is *metzitzah* an integral part of ritual circumcision? Is the circumcision invalid without this act? Must the *metzitzah* be done with the mouth?

Answer and comment: The *Mishneh Torah* of Maimonides, Karo's *Shulchan Aruch*, and others state that a *mohel* (ritual circumciser) who fails to perform *metzitzah* should be rebuked. However, the circumcision is still valid.

Traditionally, *metzitzah* has been performed by directly sucking the wound with one's mouth. The *mohel* usually rinses his mouth with alcohol first in order to avoid introducing bacteria from his oral cavity into the wound. Despite the fact that it is virtually impossible to sterilize the oral cavity by such methods, some authorities vehemently argue against a change in tradition, and insist on direct mouth sucking. Alternative methods such as interposing a short glass tube, rubber tubing, gauze pad, or the barrel of a sterile 5cc syringe are all acceptable and perfectly valid in the opinion of most authorities.

The special concerns that have arisen due to the widespread occurrence of AIDS and hepatitis are additional reasons for the meticulous observance of aseptic techniques.

Subject: *Neonatal jaundice and ritual circumcision.*

Question: What are the medical criteria for delaying a ritual circumcision because of jaundice? If a *brit* has to be postponed, must there be a seven-day minimum wait as in the case of any infant classified as ill (*choleh*)?

Answer and Comment: *Halachah* demands that a jaundiced infant not be circumcised because "one must not circumcise a child who is possibly ill since any danger to the child's life sets aside all religious requirements, for it is possible to circumcise at a later date but it is impossible to restore a life" (Talmud Shabbat 134b and *Yoreh Deah* 263:1). Maimonides explains (*Hilchot Milah* 1:17) that the jaundice referred to is "excessively yellow" (*yarok beyoter*). The author of *Shulchan Aruch* asserts that all must perforce agree that the law applies to "excessive jaundice," for such an infant is considered ill (*choleh*) because this is not the norm for newborns.

Physiologic jaundice is a "normal" state for a neonate. The qualification "excessive" means either excessive in the quantity of bilirubin or excessive in the persistence of hyperbilirubinemia for longer than normal. Recently, it has been shown (*Science* 235:1043–1045, 1987) that bilirubin may have a "beneficial" role as a physiological antioxidant. Thus bilirubin may be likened to many physiologically active molecules that are beneficial in physiologic doses but harmful at "excessive" or toxic levels.

A better understanding of physiologic jaundice associated with a more relaxed attitude toward treatment has therefore occurred. Many physicians do not put a jaundiced term baby under bilirubin lamps if he is otherwise normal, without any evidence of an ABO incompatibility, provided the bilirubin level remains less than twenty in the physiological peak at three to five days. This approach has enabled more babies to have normal early maternal and paternal bonding instead of being placed under the bilirubin lamps, naked and with covered eyes.

The *mohel* (Jewish ritual circumciser) in the past was hesitant to perform a *brit* on a yellow child, fearing that he might be ill. Thus, the *brit* would be postponed. Jewish law prohibits doing a *brit* on a baby who may have a systemic illness (i.e., sepsis), as this would put the child's life in danger. But, because of our current understanding of physiologic jaundice, *mohelim*, too, should approach jaundiced babies differently than in the past. A child with physiological jaundice should have a brit on the eighth day, even if the child is yellow, provided that there is clear evidence that the liver is properly conjugating the bilirubin as manifested by a significant spontaneous bilirubin level drop of at least 10 percent from the peak level.

It is clear that a medical opinion that delay is required is fully binding halachically. The situation that is less clear is when the physician has no objection to the circumcision but the child is frankly jaundiced. The "illness" of the child is clearly not the yellow pigment in his skin or sclerae but the failure of the liver because of its immaturity to conjugate a normal quantity of bilirubin, or the excessive amounts of bilirubin produced by hemolysis (excessive destruction of blood) as occurs in sepsis. Therefore, "cure" or restoration to good health is not to be measured by a color chart but by biochemical and/or clinical evidence that the baby's liver is now functioning properly or that the sepsis or hemolysis or other underlying cause for the jaundice has been reversed.

Most rabbinic authorities therefore emphasize that not all "yellowness" is a sign of illness requiring a seven-day wait before ritual circumcision can be performed. The early clearing of the jaundice or "yellowness" indicates that the baby was not ill but had physiologic dysfunction. When the circumcision was delayed because of doubt (saphek), as soon as the doubt is clarified, there is no need to wait seven days. If, however, there is clear evidence that the child was indeed ill—as explained above—and the basis for the increased intensity or prolonged duration of jaundice is more than just physiologic jaundice, then a seven-day waiting period is required from the time that the child is declared to be recovered from the underlying illness.

Additional Sources:

1. Chochmat Adam 149.
2. Responsa Avnei Nezer, Yoreh Deah 320.
3. Responsa Maharsham, Part 4, #120.
4. Levi, Y. Noam, Vol. 10, 5727 (1967).

DEATH AND DYING

Subject: *Informing the critically ill patient.*

Question: Must the physician inform the critically ill patient of the seriousness of the illness? Is it sufficient to inform the patient's next of kin?

Answer: In Jewish law, patients suffering from a fatal illness should be told only that they are seriously ill, but the disease should not be identified nor the true prognosis revealed if such revelation might increase the psychotrauma of the patient.

Comment: In the Jewish view, patients suffering from a fatal illness should not be so informed if there is the slightest chance that such knowledge may further impair the physical or mental well-being of the patient. Jewish ethics permit and even require that the facts concerning the true severity of the illness be withheld from the patient. The patient should be made aware that he is seriously ill so that he may be forewarned to "set his house in order," but this should be done without giving the patient a totally negative outlook. Rather, the positive side of the illness including the chances for cure, however remote, should be emphasized. Only in exceptional circumstances should the truth be divulged to the patient. Even then it should be emphasized that medical prognostications may be grossly inaccurate, lest they further reduce the morale and defense capabilities of the patient and his family. Mention of death should be avoided, if possible, lest the will to live be undermined.

Sources: *Shulchan Aruch, Yoreh Deah* 337 and 338 and the Commentary of *Shach* there, subsections 1 and 2.

Subject: *Euthanasia.*

Question: Is mercy killing allowed by Jewish law? If a patient is being maintained only through the use of a pacemaker and/or respirator, may the physician "throw the switch"?

Answer: Any form of active euthanasia is strictly prohibited by Jewish law and considered plain murder.

Comment: Judaism condemns any deliberate induction of death, and considers it an act of murder, even if the patient requests it. Life is not ours to terminate. It is therefore absolutely forbidden to administer any drug or institute any procedure that may hasten the death of the patient, unless such drugs or procedures have significant therapeutic potential. The discontinuation of instrumentation and machinery such as a respirator or cardiac pacemaker, which are specifically designed and utilized to treat critically ill patients, would be permissible only if the physician is certain that in so doing he is not interrupting life. Such a determination seems impossible for the physician to make with absolute certainty and therefore, once instituted, instrumental support of vital life processes should not be interrupted, unless and until halachic death has been established.

If the patient in extremis is in severe pain and no therapeutic protocol holds any hope for his recovery, it may be proper to withhold any *additional* nonroutine medical services, so as to permit the natural ebbing of the life forces.

Subject: *Definition of death in Jewish law.*

Question: What is the halachic definition of death?

Answer: A patient who has no evidence of either spontaneous respiration or heart action for ten minutes or more of continuous observation is considered halachically dead, provided resuscitation is deemed impossible.

Comment: The absence of spontaneous respiration and the absence of any palpable pulse are the cardinal signs for ascertaining death. A waiting period is required after spontaneous respiration and heartbeat have ceased, in order for all doubts to be set aside.

In cases such as drowning or individuals struck by lightning, resuscitation must be attempted. The same holds true for other instances where resuscitation is deemed possible.

Cerebral death (flat electroencephalogram) is *not* an acceptable criterion of death in Jewish law. *Total* cessation of all brain function as determined by the "Harvard criteria" *and* radioisotopic confirmation that the brain stem is not being perfused *is* absolute evidence that death has occurred (see following essay).

Source: *Shulchan Aruch, Yoreh Deah 370.*

PHYSIOLOGIC DECAPITATION AS A DEFINITION OF DEATH IN JUDAISM*

Introduction

The modern era of human heart transplantation, which began late in 1967, initiated intense debate about the moral, religious, and legal issues relating to life and death and especially the definition of death. The traditional definition of death as reflected in *Black's Law Dictionary* is the "total stoppage of the circulation of the blood, and the cessation of the animal and vital functions consequent thereon, such as respiration, pulsation. . . ." With the advent of heart transplantation, this definition of death became inadequate and a new definition of death, so-called brain death, evolved. Brain death is now socially acceptable and legislatively sanctioned throughout most of the civilized world.

In a classic 1968 article on brain death[1], an Ad Hoc Committee of the Harvard Medical School recommended four criteria: unreceptivity and unresponsivity, no movements, no reflexes, and a flat electroencephalogram. This paper was reprinted as a "Landmark Article" in 1984[2] with an accompanying perspective editorial[3], which states:

> The Harvard Committee report likely spawned more medicolegal discussion and action than any other publication. Almost every legal entity has had to deal with this new concept of death, and most medical standards for death of the brain originate, with some modifications, from the criteria set forth in this article. The prescience of this committee has become even more obvious as hundreds of clinical observations have borne out the diagnostic value of their clearly stated clinical rules.

*Reprinted with permission from the *Journal of Halacha and Contemporary Society* #17, Spring 1989 (Pesach 5749), pp. 14–31.

In 1981, the President's Commission for the Study of Ethical Problems in Medicine and Biomedical and Behavioral Research published its report that defined death.[4] This definition was approved by the American Bar Association, the American Medical Association, and many other organizations and prominent individuals. The recommended proposal was the following:

> An individual who has sustained either (a) irreversible cessation of circulatory and respiratory functions, or (b) irreversible cessation of all functions of the entire brain, including the brain stem, is dead. A determination of death must be made in accordance with accepted medical standards.

The duration of time for observation has not been settled. The Harvard Ad Hoc Committee stated "all of the above tests shall be repeated at least 24 hours later with no change." The President's Commission recommended an observation period of six hours if confirmatory tests are available and twelve hours if they are not. For anoxic brain damage, the Commission stated that twenty-four hours of observation is generally desirable for ascertainment of brain death but that this period may be reduced if a test shows cessation of cerebral blood flow or if an electroencephalogram shows electrocerebral silence (i.e., a flat tracing) in an adult patient without drug intoxication, hypothermia, or shock.

At present, most statutes and judicial opinions accept the extension of the definition of death first introduced by the Harvard Ad Hoc Committee and recognize that death can be accurately demonstrated either on the traditional grounds of irreversible cessation of heart and lung functions or on the basis of irreversible loss of all functions of the entire brain. This recognition is codified in the Uniform Determination of Death Act, which does not specify diagnostic tests or medical procedures required to determine death but leaves the medical profession free to make use of new medical knowledge and diagnostic advances as they become available. The determination of death must thus be made in accordance with accepted medical standards.

In New York State, the governor in 1984 appointed a Task Force on Life and the Law, which published its recommendations on the Determination of Death in July 1986. The Task Force suggested that the New York State Department of Health promulgate a regulation which establishes that an individual is dead when the individual has suffered either (a) irreversible cessation of respiratory and circulatory functions or (b) irreversible cessation of all functions of the entire brain, including the brain stem. On June 18, 1987, the State Hospital Review and Planning Council adopted a regulation recognizing the total and irreversible cessation of brain function as a basis for determining death in New York State. Shortly thereafter, the Department of Health amended its regulations to include this standard so that either the brain death standard or the circulatory or respiratory standard may be relied on to determine that death has occurred.

The brain death standard applies to hospital and nursing home patients who have lost all brain function and whose breathing and circulation are artificially maintained. Under the standard, patients like Karen Ann Quinlan, who have brain capacity and the ability to regulate basic functions such as heartbeat and respiration, are considered alive.

It is of paramount importance not to confuse brain death with other forms of irreversible brain damage, particularly the permanent vegetative state. At present, a patient in such a state is alive according to all legal, moral, medical, and religious definitions. Such a patient is certainly not dead in the medical or legal sense and his organs may not be removed for transplantation until death has been established by either classic irreversible cardiorespiratory criteria or by irreversible brain stem death criteria.

Does Judaism Recognize Brain Death?

There is at present an intense debate among rabbinic authorities as to whether or not Jewish law (halachah) recognizes brain death as a definition of death. It is our thesis that the answer is affirmative. The classic definition of death in Judaism as found in the Talmud and Codes of Jewish Law is the absence of spontaneous respiration in a person who appears dead (i.e., shows no movements and is unresponsive to all stimuli). The absence of hypothermia or drug overdose must be ascertained because these conditions can result in depression of the respiratory center with absence of spontaneous respiration and even heartbeat. If resuscitation is deemed possible, no matter how remote the chance, it must be attempted.

Jewish writings provide considerable evidence for the thesis that the brain and the brain stem control all bodily functions including respiration and cardiac activity. It, therefore, follows that if there is irreversible total cessation of all brain function including that of the brain stem, the person is dead, even though there may still be some transient spontaneous cardiac activity. Brain function is divided into higher cerebral activities and the vegetative functions of the vital centers of the brain stem. A criterion of death based on higher cerebral death alone is ethically and morally unacceptable. If a person is decapitated, his heart and lungs may still function for a brief period of time but that person is obviously dead at the moment the brain and brain stem are severed from the remainder of the body. If one can medically establish that there is total cessation of all brain function including the brain stem, the patient is as if "physiologically decapitated."

There are a number of objective tests that can evaluate the viability of the brain stem. These include isotope and other angiography (blood flow) studies, the apnea test, evoked potential studies, and others. Brain stem death may be the preferable definition of death in Judaism since it is irreversible. Brain stem death confirms bodily death in a patient with absence of spontaneous respiration who may still have a heartbeat. We will provide support for our position from ancient and recent Jewish sources.

Classic Definition of Death in Jewish Law

The definition of death in Jewish law is first mentioned in the fifth century Babylonian Talmud which enumerates circumstances under which one may desecrate the Sabbath.[5]

> every danger to human life suspends the [laws of the] Sabbath. If debris [of a collapsing building] falls on someone and it is doubtful whether he is there or whether he is not there, or if it is doubtful whether he is an Israelite or a heathen, one must probe the heap of the debris for his sake [even on the Sabbath]. If one finds him alive, one should remove the debris, but if he is dead, one leaves him there [until after the Sabbath].

The Talmud then comments as follows:[6]

How far does one search [to ascertain whether he is dead or alive]? Until [one reaches] his nose. Some say: Up to his heart. . . . life manifests itself primarily through the nose, as it is written: *In whose nostrils was the breath of the spirit of life.*[7]

The renowned biblical and talmudic commentator Rashi explains that if no air emanates from his nostrils, he is certainly dead. Rashi further explains that some people suggest the heart be examined for signs of life, but the respiration test is considered of greatest import.

The rule is codified by Maimonides as follows:[8]

If, upon examination, no sign of breathing can be detected at the nose, the victim must be left where he is [until after the Sabbath] because he is already dead.

The universally accepted code of Jewish law by Joseph Karo, known as *Shulchan Aruch*, states:[9]

Even if the victim was found so severely injured that he cannot live for more than a short while, one must probe [the debris] until one reaches his nose. If one cannot detect signs of respiration at the nose, then he is certainly dead whether the head was uncovered first or whether the feet were uncovered first.

Neither Maimonides nor Karo require examination of the heart. Cessation of respiration seems to be the determining physical sign for the ascertainment of death.

Another pertinent passage found in Karo's code states as follows:[10]

If a woman is sitting on the birthstool [i.e., about to give birth] and she dies, one brings a knife on the Sabbath, even through a public domain, and one incises her womb and removes the fetus, since one might find it alive.

Rabbi Moses Isserles, known as *Rama*, adds to this statement:[11]

However, today we do not conduct ourselves according to this [rule] even during the week [i.e., even *not* on the Sabbath] because we are not competent to recognize precisely the moment of maternal death.

Several commentators explain that Isserles is concerned that perhaps the mother only fainted, and incising her abdomen might kill her. Maimonides, five centuries earlier, had already raised the problem of fainting complicating the recognition of death when he stated: "Whosoever closes the eyes of the dying while the soul is about to depart is shedding blood. One should wait a while: perhaps he is only in a swoon."[12]

Both Maimonides and Isserles, however, agree that the talmudic description of death, for all practical purposes, is the absence or cessation of respiration.

Recent Rabbinic Writings on the Definition of Death

The classic Jewish legal definition says that death is established when spontaneous respiration ceases. Rabbi Moses Schreiber asserts that if a person is motionless like an inanimate stone and has no palpable pulse either in the neck or at the wrist, and also has no spontaneous respiration, his soul has certainly departed, but one should wait a short while to fulfill the requirement of Maimonides, who was concerned that the patient may only be in a swoon.[13] Rabbi Sholom Mordechai Schwadron states that if any sign of life is observed in limbs other than the heart and lungs, the apparent absence of spontaneous respiration is not conclusive in establishing death.[14]

On the other hand, Rav Isaac Yehuda Unterman, addressing the Eleventh Congress on Jewish Law in Jerusalem in August 1968, stated that one is dead when one has stopped breathing. Thus, most talmudic and post-talmudic sages agree that the absence of spontaneous respiration is the only sign needed to ascertain death. A minority would also require cessation of heart action. Thus, a patient who has stopped breathing, says Unterman, and whose heart is not beating is considered dead in Jewish law.[15]

Rav Eliezer Yehuda Waldenberg also defines death as the cessation of respiration and cardiac activity.[16] One must use all available medical means to ascertain with certainty that respiratory and cardiac functions have indeed ceased. A flat electroencephalogram in the face of a continued heartbeat is not an acceptable finding by itself to pronounce a patient dead. Even after death has been established one should wait a while before moving the deceased.

Rav Immanuel Jakobovits states, in part, that "the classic definition of death as given in the Talmud and Codes is acceptable today and correct. However, this would be set aside in cases where competent medical opinion deems any prospects of resuscitation, however remote, at all feasible."[17]

Rav J. David Bleich traces the Jewish legal attitude concerning the definition of death from talmudic through recent rabbinic times.[18] In his opinion, brain death and irreversible coma are not acceptable definitions of death insofar as Jewish law is concerned, since the sole criterion of death accepted by Jewish law is total cessation of both cardiac and respiratory activity long enough to make resuscitation impossible. Bleich also discusses the various time-of-death statutes already enacted into law in many states in this country and statutes being contemplated by other states.[19] He expresses the hope that provisions allowing for exemption from legislated definitions of death for reasons of conscience will be written into such statutes in order to preserve civil and religious liberties.

Total Brain Death in Judaism

The position that complete and permanent absence of any brain-related vital bodily function is recognized as death in Jewish law is supported by Hagaon Rav Moshe Feinstein[20] whose responsum on heart transplantation begins with a discussion of decapitation. Feinstein quotes Maimonides[21] who states that a person who is decapitated imparts ritual defilement to others because he is considered dead even though one or more limbs of the body may yet move spastically, temporarily. The situation is comparable to the severed tail from a lizard which may still quiver temporarily but is certainly not alive.[22] Feinstein asserts that "someone whose head has been severed—even if the head and the body shake spastically—that person is legally dead." The requirement of Maimonides cited earlier in this essay to wait a while when death is thought to have occurred (i.e., when the patient has no spontaneous respiratory activity), according to Feinstein, is to differentiate between true death and the situation "where the illness is so severe that the patient has no strength to breathe." Since only a few minutes of absent breathing is compatible with life, if the patient is observed for fifteen minutes with no spontaneous respirations, he is legally dead (unless a potentially reversible cause of respiratory absence is present such as hypothermia or drug overdose).

In the same responsum Feinstein prohibits heart transplantation if the donor's heart is removed before total brain death has occurred. The final paragraph of Feinstein's responsum states that it is both a meritorious or pious deed as well as a commandment (Hebrew: mitzvah) for the family of a deceased person to allow the donation of one or more organs for transplantation into recipients whose lives would thereby be saved. The presence of any spontaneous respiratory activity, however, indicates that a person is still alive and no matter what the clinical neurological picture, the patient may not be considered dead for any purpose including organ transplantation.

The above responsum is dated 1968 (5728 in the Hebrew calendar). Another Feinstein responsum dated two years later[23] amplifies the Jewish legal definition of death. Feinstein reiterates the error of physicians who diagnose death when the patient has no cerebral function but is still breathing spontaneously. This responsum also prohibits heart transplantation as murder of the recipient because his life is thereby shortened since (at that time) the success of cardiac transplantation in prolonging life had not been demonstrated.

On May 24, 1976, Rav Feinstein sent a letter to the Honorable Herbert J. Miller, who was Chairman of the New York State Assembly's Committee on Health, relevant to Assembly Bill 414Q/A concerning the determination of death. In his letter Feinstein said:

> The sole criterion of death is the total cessation of spontaneous respiration.
>
> In a patient presenting the clinical picture of death, i.e., no signs of life such as movement or response to stimuli, the total cessation of independent respiration is an absolute proof that death had occurred. This interruption of spontaneous breathing must be for a sufficient length of time for resuscitation to be impossible (approximately 15 min.).
>
> If such a "clinically dead" patient is on a respirator it is forbidden to interrupt the respirator. However, when the respirator requires servicing, the services may be withheld while the patient is carefully and continuously monitored to detect any signs of independent breathing no matter how feeble. If such breathing motions do not occur, it is a certainty that he is dead. If they do occur the respirator shall be immediately restarted.

A more recent responsum of Rav Feinstein, dated 1976,[24] further supports the acceptability of "physiologic decapitation" as an absolute definition of death. Feinstein again reiterates the classic definition of death as being the total irreversible cessation of respiration. He then states that if by injecting a substance into the vein of a patient, physicians can ascertain that there is no circulation to the brain, meaning no connection between the brain and the rest of the body, that patient is legally dead in Judaism because he is equivalent to a decapitated person. Where the test is available, continues Feinstein, it should be used.

We interpret Rav Feinstein's written responsa to indicate that Jewish law clearly recognizes that death occurs before all organs cease functioning. Cellular death follows organismal death. Jewish law defines death as an organismal phenomenon involving dissociation of the correlative or coordinating activities of the body and not as individual organ death.

The continued beating of the heart is of no *halachic* import. In the case of the Talmud where the patient is buried under debris, the interest focuses on any sign of residual life to warrant desecrating the Sabbath to dig him out. It has no relevance to a patient lying in an intensive care unit whose every function is monitored and whose status is open to full evaluation. In such a case, the issue is truly one of definition, not confirmation.

Based on the Feinstein position cited above, one of us (MDT) introduced the concept of physiologic decapitation as an acceptable definition of death in Judaism even if cardiac function has not ceased.[25]

The thesis at that time was:[26]

> that absent heartbeat or pulse was not considered a significant factor in ascertaining death in any early religious source. Furthermore, the scientific fact that cellular death does not occur at the same time as the death of the human being is well recognized in the earliest biblical sources. The twitching of a lizard's amputated tail or the death throes of a decapitated man were never considered residual life but simply manifestations of cellular life that continued after death of the entire organism had occurred. In the situation of decapitation, death can be defined or determined by the decapitated state itself as recognized in the Talmud and the Code of Laws. Complete destruction of the brain, which includes loss of all integrative, regulatory, and other functions

of the brain, can be considered physiological decapitation and thus a determinant per se of death of the person.

Loss of the ability to breathe spontaneously is a crucial criterion for determining whether complete destruction of the brain has occurred. Earliest biblical sources recognized the ability to breathe independently as a prime index of life . . . destruction of the entire brain or brain death, and only that, is consonant with biblical pronouncements on what constitutes an acceptable definition of death, i.e., a patient who has all the appearances of lifelessness and who is no longer breathing spontaneously. Patients with irreversible total destruction of the brain fulfill this definition even if heart action and circulation are artificially maintained.

Thus, if it can be definitely demonstrated that all brain functions including brain stem function have ceased, the patient is legally dead in Jewish law because he is equated with a decapitated individual whose heart may still be beating. Brain stem function can be accurately evaluated by radionuclide cerebral angiography at the patient's bedside.[27–30] This test is a stress-free, simple, safe, highly specific, and highly reliable indicator of absence of blood flow to the entire brain, thus confirming total irreversible brain death. "The absence of cerebral blood flow is presently considered the most reliable ancillary test in diagnosing brain death."[31] Other presently used tests to confirm brain death are the apnea test,[32–33] evoked potentials,[34] transcranial Doppler studies,[35] xenon-enhanced computed tomography,[36] and digital subtraction angiography.[37] The electroencephalogram is not a reliable index for the establishment of brain death since it only indicates activity of the cerebral cortex and does not clarify brain stem function at all. Furthermore, electroencephalographic activity can be observed for many hours after "brain death" in both adults[38] and children.[39]

Extensive recent medical reviews confirm that cessation of brain flow as measured by radioisotope techniques is invariably accompanied by signs of brain cell lysis. This evidence of cellular decay, although confirmable only at post-mortem examination, is an absolute criterion of death despite the beating heart. The heart is not dependent for its stimulation on brain function. A heart completely removed from the body continues to beat as long as its nutrition is maintained. Rav Feinstein is firmly of the opinion that the sole criterion of death in a patient who gives the clinical impression of death is cessation of spontaneous respiration. "Clinical impression of death" means "if he resembles a dead person, that is to say he does not move any of his limbs."[40]

When a patient is on a respirator and gives all the evidence of having died, i.e., meets the Harvard criteria, he is not "brain dead"— a confusing term—but is dead as evidenced, first and foremost, by cessation of independent respiration. In addition, a careful check must be made that he meets the reservation that he appear clinically dead. This requirement is met in the fullest and most absolute measure by total unreceptivity, unresponsiveness, absence of all movements, absent cephalic reflexes, fixed dilated pupils, and persistence of all these findings for at least a twenty-four hour period in the absence of intoxicants or hypothermia. These are the Harvard criteria.

Thus, the only valid definition of death is brain death. The classic "respiratory and circulatory death" is in reality brain death. Irreversible respiratory arrest is indicative of brain death. A brain dead person is a physiologically decapitated individual. The requirement of Maimonides to "wait a while" to confirm that the patient is dead is that amount of time it takes after the heart and lungs stop until the brain dies, i.e., a few minutes. Until the brain dies, one must attempt to restart the heart and the respiration of a non-breathing patient. If the heart and lung function are rapidly restored the patient may suffer no neurological deficits. Thus, we see that Jewish law defines death as brain death. There are a number of objective tests now available that can evaluate the viability of the brain stem. A simple, non-stressful test is the radionuclide blood flow study described above. This test does not violate the prohibition against unnecessarily stressing the patient in any way and has been shown to be nearly 100% accurate.

Another strong proof for our thesis that brain death is the Jewish legal definition of death is found in Karo's Code of Jewish Law.[41] The author describes individuals "who are considered dead even though they are still alive" to include those whose necks have been broken and those whose bodies "are torn on the back like a fish." These people are considered dead in that they impart ritual defilement and render their wives widows even though they may still have spastic or convulsive movements and even have heartbeats. The reason is that the connection between the brain and the body has been severed by the severance of the spinal cord or by the severance of the blood supply to the brain. It thus seems clear that death of the brain is the legal definition of death in *halachah*.

The fifteenth century commentator, Yehudah Aryeh of Modinah, who was Rabbi in Venice and known by the pen name of *Omar Haboneh*, states:[42]

> All [Rabbis] agree that the fundamental source of life is in the brain. Therefore, if one examines the nose first which is an organ of servitude of the brain and there is no [spontaneous] respiration, none of them [i.e., the Rabbis] doubt that life has departed from the brain.

Further support for our position can be deduced from the talmudic precedent[43] which is codified in Jewish law[44] about the woman who dies in labor and the unborn fetus is still alive. As cited earlier, since the woman may only be in coma and not dead "because we are not competent to recognize precisely the moment of maternal death,"[45] we do not perform an immediate cesarian section to try to save the unborn child because the comatose but alive mother might be killed thereby. However, where death is certain, as for example if the mother was accidentally decapitated, an immediate cesarian section is required[46] although individual limbs or organs of the mother may still exhibit muscular spasms.

Rav Nachum Rabinowitz[47] quotes Maimonides[48] who explains that the organism is no longer considered to be alive "when the power of locomotion that is spread throughout the limbs does not originate in one center, but is independently spread throughout the body." Obviously, continues Rabinowitz, "the definition of death depends upon the availiability of more sophisticated techniques of resuscitation." Again citing Maimonides,[49] Rabinowitz concludes that the applicability of such methods and the consequent decision as to the onset of death is determined according to the judgment of the physicians. We believe that the sophisticated medical techniques described above including radionuclide angiography can definitively establish the absence of any possibility of resuscitation, equating such a physiologically decapitated patient with the hypothetical case of the decapitated woman whose death is confirmed by her decapitated status even though she may still exhibit muscular spasms.

In a later publication,[50] Rabinowitz quotes another citation from Maimonides[51] as follows: "If a person's neck is broken . . . or if his back is torn like a fish or if he is decapitated or if he is hemisected at the abdomen, he imparts ritual defilement [because he is dead] even if one of his organs is still shaking." From here it can be concluded, continues Rabinowitz, that if the controlling center which unifies all the activities of the organs is nullified (i.e., dead), the movement of a single organ is meaningless and does not indicate that the person (i.e., the organism) is alive.

We are aware of opposition to our point of view. Rav Aaron Soloveichik considers our position to be a serious misinterpretation of Jewish law.[52] One of us (MDT) effectively replied to that criticism.[53] We maintain our position, however, that total and irreversible cessation of all brain function as determined by the Harvard criteria is equivalent to total destruction of the brain and hence, tantamount to functional or physiological decapitation which in Judaism is equated with death.

Conclusion

Judaism is guided by the concepts of the supreme sanctity of human life, and of the dignity of man created in the image of God. The preservation of human life in Judaism is a divine commandment. Jewish law requires the physician to do everything in his power to prolong life, but prohibits the use of measures that prolong the act of dying. The value attached to human life in Judaism is far greater than that in Christian tradition or in Anglo-Saxon common law. To save a life, all Jewish religious laws are automatically suspended, the only exceptions being idolatry, murder, and forbidden sexual relations such as incest. In Jewish law and moral teaching, the value of human life is infinite and beyond measure, so that any part of life—even if only an hour or a second—is of precisely the same worth as seventy years of it.

When does life end is an issue which is presently being actively discussed. All rabbis agree that the classic definition of death in Judaism is the absence of spontaneous respiration in a patient with no bodily motion. A brief waiting period of a few minutes to a half hour after breathing has ceased is also required. If hypothermia or drug overdose which can result in depression of the respiratory center with absence of spontaneous respiration and even heartbeat are present, this classic definition of death is insufficient. Hence, wherever resuscitation is deemed possible, no matter how remote the chance, it must be attempted unless there are ethical and moral considerations for cessation of all therapy. Brain death is a criterion for confirming death in a patient who already has irreversible absence of spontaneous respiration. The situation of decapitation, where immediate death is assumed even if the heart may still be briefly beating, is certainly equated with organismal death. Whether or not total, irreversible brain stem death, as evidenced by sophisticated medical testing, is the Jewish legal equivalent of decapitation is presently a matter of debate in rabbinic circles. We are of the opinion that it is.

Although the topic of organ transplantation in Judaism is beyond the scope of this essay, vital organ transplants are directly related to the definition of death, particularly brain death. Thus, when a patient is dead, it is at least an act of loving kindness and perhaps even a moral obligation for the next of kin to allow the transplantation of organs from the deceased into living persons dying of organ failure whose lives can be saved by an organ transplant. Where a patient's life is at stake, such organ transplantation is permissible and perhaps even mandated, but consent from the donor or next of kin should be obtained prior to transplantation. The biblical injunctions regarding the donor which prohibit desecration of the dead, deriving benefit from the dead, and delaying the burial of the dead are suspended for the greater consideration of saving the recipient's life. The donor must be dead before any organ may be removed for transplantation. The age, sex, race, religion, or ethnic background of both donor and recipient are irrelevant.

REFERENCES

1. A definition of irreversible coma. Report of the Ad Hoc Committee of the Harvard Medical School to Examine the Definition of Brain Death. *J.A.M.A.* 1968; 205:337–350.
2. *Ibid. J.A.M.A.* 1984; 252:677–679.
3. Joynt RJ, A new look at death. *J.A.M.A.* 1984; 252:680–682.
4. President's Commission for the Study of Ethical Problems in Medicine and Biomedical and Behavioral Research, *Defining Death: Medical, Legal and Ethical Issues in the Determination of Death.* Government Printing Office, 1981.
5. Tractate Yoma 8:6–7.
6. *Ibid.* folio 85a.
7. Genesis 7:22.
8. Maimonides M, *Mishneh Torah* (Code of Maimonides), *Hilchot Shabbat,* (Laws of the Sabbath) 2:19.
9. Karo J, *Shulchan Aruch* (Code of Jewish Law), Section *Orach Chayim* 329:4.
10. *Ibid.* 330:5.
11. Isserles M, Glossary on Karo's *Shulchan Aruch,* Section *Orach Chayim* 330:5.
12. Maimonides M, *Mishneh Torah, Hilchot Avel* (Laws of Mourning) 4:5.
13. Schreiber M, Responsa *Chatam Sofer,* Section *Yoreh Deah,* No. 338.
14. Schwadron, SM, Responsa *Maharsham.* Vol. 4, Sect. 6, No. 124.
15. Unterman IY, Points of Halachah in Heart Transplantation. *Noam* 1970; 13:1–9.
16. Waldenberg EY, Responsa *Tzitz Eliezer.* Vol. 9, No. 46 and Vol. 10, No. 25:4.
17. Jakobovits I. Personal communication, August 1, 1968.
18. Bleich JD, *Contemporary Halakhic Problems.* New York, KTAV, 1977, pp. 372–393.
19. Bleich JD, Time of death legislation. *Tradition* 1977; 16:130–139.
20. Feinstein M, Responsa *Iggrot Moshe,* Section *Yoreh Deah,* Part 2, No. 174.
21. Maimonides M, *Mishneh Torah, Hilchot Tumat Met* (Laws concerning ritual defilement by the dead) 1:15.
22. Babylonian Talmud, Tractate Oholot 1:6.
23. Feinstein M, Responsa *Iggrot Moshe,* Section *Yoreh Deah,* Part 2, No. 146.
24. Feinstein M, Responsa *Iggrot Moshe,* Section *Yoreh Deah,* Part 3, No. 132.
25. Tendler MD, Cessation of brain function. Ethical implications in termi-

nal care and organ transplants. *Annals NY Acad. Sci.* 1978; *315*:394–497.

26. Veith FJ, Fein JM, Tendler MD, et al., Brain death. I. A status report of medical and ethical considerations. *J.A.M.A.* 1977; *238*:1651–1655.

27. Korein J, Braunstein P, George A, et al., Brain death. I. Angiographic correlation with the radioisotopic bolus technique for evaluation of critical deficit of cerebral flow. *Ann. Neurol.* 1977; *2*:195–205.

28. Tsai SH, Cranford RE, Rockswold G, Koehler S, Cerebral radionuclide angiography. *J.A.M.A.* 1982; *248*:591–592.

29. Schwartz JA, Baxter J, Brill D, Diagnosis of brain death in children by radionuclide cerebral imaging. *Pediatrics* 1982; *73*:14–18.

30. Goodman JM, Heck LL, Moore BD, Confirmation of brain death with portable isotope angiography. A review of 204 consecutive cases. *Neurosurgery* 1985; *16*:492–497.

31. Alvarez LA, Lipton RB, Hirschfeld A, et al., Brain death determination by angiography in the setting of a skull defect. *Arch. Neurol.* 1988; *45*:225–227.

32. Ropper AH, Kennedy SK, Russell L, Apnea testing in the diagnosis of brain death: clinical and physiological observations. *J. Neurosurg.* 1981; *55*:942–946.

33. Rowland TW, Donnelly JH, Jackson AH, Apnea documentation for determination of brain death in children. *Pediatrics* 1984; *74*:505–508.

34. Trojaborg W, Jorgensen EO, Evoked cortical potentials in patients with "isolectric" EEG. *Electroencephalogr. Clin. Neurophysiol.* 1973; *35*:301–309.

35. Ropper AH, Kehne SM, Wechsler L, Transcranial Doppler in brain death. *Neurology* 1987; *37*:1733–1735.

36. Darby J, Yonas H, Brenner RP, Brainstem death with persistent EEG activity. Evaluation by xenon-enhanced computed tomography. *Critical Care Med.* 1987; *15*:519–521.

37. Tan WS, Wilbur AC, Jafar JJ, et al., Brain death. Use of dynamic CT and intravenous digital subtraction angiography. *Amer. J. Neurorad.* 1987; *8*:123–125.

38. Grigg MM, Kelly MA, Celesia GG, et al., Electroencephalographic activity after brain death. *Arch. Neurol.* 1987; *44*:948–954.

39. Ashwal S, Schneider S, Failure of electroencephalography to diagnose brain death in comatose children. *Ann. Neurol.* 1979; *6*:512–517.

40. Rashi's talmudic commentary on tractate Yoma 85a (s.v. *ad hechan*).

41. Karo J, *Shulchan Aruch*, Section *Yoreh Deah* 370.

42. Modinah YA, Commentary *Omar Haboneh* in Jacob Habib's *Eeyun Yaakov*, Tractate Yoma 85a.

43. Tractate Arachin 7:1.

44. Karo J, *Shulchan Aruch*, Section *Orach Chayim* 330:5.

45. Isserles M, Glossary on Karo's *Shulchan Aruch*, Section *Orach Chayim* 330:5.
46. Reischer J, Responsa *Shevut Yaakov*. Vol. 1, No. 13.
47. Rabinowitz N, What is the *halakhah* for organ transplants? *Tradition* (New York) 1968; 9:20–27.
48. Maimonides M, *Mishnah Commentary*, Tractate Oholot 1:6.
49. Maimonides M, *Mishneh Torah*, *Hilchot Rotze'ach* (Laws of Murder) 2:8.
50. Rabinowitz NE, Sign of life: a single organism. *Techumin*, Zomet, Alon Shevut, Gush Etzion, Israel, Vol. 8, 1987 (5747), pp. 442–443.
51. Maimonides M, *Mishneh Torah*, *Hilchot Tumat Met* 1:15.
52. Soloveichik A, Jewish law and time of death. *J.A.M.A.* 1978; *240*:109.
53. Tendler MD, Jewish law and time of death. *J.A.M.A.* 1978; *240*:109.

Anencephalics ("brain absent") and "brain death"

Brain Absent: The Problem

Brain absent is a relatively new term in medical ethics. It is a term used to make more acceptable the use of anencephalic infants as organ donors. By equating brain dead with brain absent, one denies the humanhood of the patient. Brain absent is a term used by proponents of offering organs for transplantation from anencephalic infants at birth by declaring them brain dead because they have no brain. However, such babies have a brain stem and often breathe independently at birth. Therefore, in Judaism, an anencephalic newborn is not brain dead, since he breathes on his own. We have an absolutely accurate definition of brain death and the anencephalic does not fit that definition. "Brain absent" is a euphemistic term to make the unacceptable palatable.

If one equates brain absent in the presence of independent respiration with brain death, the next step will be to equate loss of cerebral function in the presence of independent respiration with brain death. In fact, courts in several jurisdictions of the United States have already upheld the removal or withholding of fluids and nutrition from chronic or persistent vegetative state patients who have no cerebral or cognitive brain function yet whose hearts, lungs, kidneys, and other organs are functioning independently. Shall we offer such patients as organ farms not because they are brain dead but because they are nonfunctional in society? This is the "slippery slope" in societal ethics. The unthinkable is reality today.

It is our position that a patient who breathes independently is alive and entitled to all the care and concern of our society. An ethical society is defined by the degree of care and concern it shows to its most helpless citizens. There is no more helpless a person than a permanent vegetative state patient.

A related issue beyond the scope of this presentation is the potential or actual lack of sufficient resources for society to pay for all the care for all its citizens. A prominent bioethicist and director of the Hastings Center[1] proposes that the cost of health care for the elderly is so high that we should stop giving life-prolonging therapy to the old. If we cannot afford to provide medical care for everybody, who should get what? Priority decisions are forcing us to play God. This topic may in the near future require triage decisions that are yet unthinkable.

Brain Absent in Halachah

Brain absence presents a unique challenge in *halachah*. One point of view is that an anencephalic is considered a nonviable abortus (*nefel*) and its organs can be taken at birth for transplantation. We believe that an anencephalic or brain absent newborn and a patient with cerebral dysfunction such as a permanent vegetative state are both viewed in Jewish law as alive in that they both breathe independently. We have no other definition in *halachah* to differentiate the living from the dead.

Since there is no direct reference in Torah literature to an anencephalic newborn, the question one can pose is the following: is there a *halachic* basis for the lack of humanhood of a deformed newborn baby who is breathing independently? We believe the answer is affirmative. The Talmud[2] asserts as follows:

> For a seven months' infant [i.e., one born after seven months of pregnancy] one may desecrate the Sabbath, but for an eight months' infant one may not desecrate the Sabbath [for the Rabbis held that such could not possibly live; hence there is no point in descrating the Sabbath on its behalf]. . . . An eight months' infant is like a stone, i.e,. nonviable and may not be handled, but his mother bends [over] and suckles him because of the danger.

Rashi[3] explains the danger: "because her breasts are full of milk and would cause her to become ill" if she is not eased of her milk, i.e., danger to the mother. *Tosafot*[4] adds that today all infants may be handled on the Sabbath because we are not expert enough to recognize which is an eighth or a ninth month infant, provided the infant has hairs and nails, i.e., signs of maturity.

The same talmudic discussion occurs elsewhere in the Talmud[5] where it states that an eight month child is like a stone [i.e., nonviable] and it is forbidden to move him [on the Sabbath]; only his mother may bend over him and nurse him because of the danger.

Here, Rashi[6] explains "because of danger to both the infant and the mother," the mother because she might contract a serious illness from the excess of milk in her breasts and the infant because he might die of starvation before his time. *Tosafot*[7] adds that if the baby is fully developed and shows signs of maturity such as nails and hairs, it is permitted to handle him on the Sabbath and he is not considered like a nonviable abortus. Rashi in tractate Shabbat seems to be concerned only with danger to the mother whereas in tractate Yebamot Rashi has a dual concern for both baby and mother.

The talmudic commentary known as *Bigdei Yesha* explains the commentary of Mordechai ben Hillel Ashkenazi, known simply as *Mordechai*,[8] and indicates that there is concern for a prematurely born infant even though it has not yet achieved humanhood. Because it is not yet human, it is forbidden to handle it on the Sabbath or desecrate the Sabbath on its behalf, but one must do whatever is possible to preserve its life. Furthermore, says this commentator, if the baby was born deformed after eight and a half months of gestation and survived for two weeks, it is considered like a full term infant on whose behalf the Sabbath must be desecrated if its life is in danger.

There is thus a unique status for a deformed baby who is born prematurely in that it does not have humanhood, is not yet alive, and *halachah* prohibits its handling on the Sabbath. Maturity, however, even in the presence of deformity, entitles the baby to the full protection of *halachah* and the Sabbath must be desecrated on its behalf. Therefore, a full term or mature anencephalic newborn who is breathing independently may not be killed at birth to harvest its organs.

There is an extensive rabbinic literature[9] covering the status of the eight month infant, including recent responsa[10], and the interested reader is referred there for additional discussion of this topic. A most interesting responsum as to whether or not a deformed baby born comatose imparts ritual defilement to a *kohen* (priest) is that of Rabbi Itzila Ponevezer[11] who writes that "a deformed newborn who is still alive has the status of flesh [i.e., not alive] in certain respects but in other respects is considered alive." Whenever the *halachah* requires a person to be alive, this deformed newborn is not dead. The eight month infant seems to be in an intermediary state, neither alive nor dead. To allow desecration of the Sabbath for danger to life, we require a living person, and the eight month infant is not alive. To remove organs for transplantation requires that the donor be dead, but an eight month infant is not dead. Therefore, it is prohibited to do anything that may hasten its death.

Thus, an anencephalic newborn with independent respiration cannot be used at birth as an organ donor because it is not yet dead. But there seems to be no objection in Jewish law to transplanting organs from an anencephalic baby once it no longer has spontaneous respirations and is declared dead. From the practical standpoint, it is necessary to artificially ventilate the baby when it is no longer able to do so by itself in order to maintain organ perfusion until the transplantation procedure can be carried out.

If it is true, as claimed by many neurologists, that an anencephalic newborn feels no pain, since pain is interpreted by higher brain centers that such a baby is lacking, it seems permissible in halachah to attach a respirator and maintain an anencephalic infant until it is declared brain dead by the classic criteria described above, e.g., absent spontaneous respirations after one or more ten-minute apnea tests. Then its organs may be removed and transplanted into one or more recipients whose lives would thereby be saved. Without imposing any stress or pain on the patient, our prime concern is the saving of lives. The parents of the anencephalic child may also feel a sense of accomplishment in that some good came of their tragedy.

Such permissibility to use organs of brain dead anencephalic infants for transplantation does not extend, however, to permanent vegetative state patients. Such patients may not be placed on a respirator solely in order to serve as organ donors if there is pain or discomfort involved. One may not use one patient in this way in the servitude of another. God said:[12] *For it is to Me that the people of Israel are servants; they are My servants.* Man is in God's servitude. Man cannot demand another person in his service.

REFERENCES

1. Callahan D, *Setting Limits: Medical Goals in an Aging Society*: New York, Simon and Schuster, 1987.
2. Shabbat 135a.
3. Commentary of Rashi, Shabbat 135a; *s.v. mipney hasakanah*.
4. Commentary of Tosafot, Shabbat 135a; *s.v. ben shemonah*.
5. Yebamot 80a and 80b.
6. Commentary of Rashi, Yebamot 80b; *s.v. mipney hasakanah*.
7. Commentary of Tosafot, Yebamot 80b; *s.v. vehoh tanya*.
8. Commentary of Mordechai as explained by *Bigdei Yesha*, Shabbat 135a (p. 152 in the standard editions of the Talmud).
9. Karo J, *Shulchan Aruch, Yoreh Deah* 266:11 and 305:22–23.
10. Schreiber M, Responsa *Chatam Sofer, Yoreh Deah*, Nos. 247 and 324.
11. Ponevezer I, Responsa *Zecher Yitzchok*, No. 67.
12. Leviticus 25:55.

Subject: *Autopsy in Jewish law.*

Question: When, if ever, is an autopsy permitted in Jewish law (*halachah*)? How must it be conducted? When is it permissible for a physician to ask consent from the next of kin for an autopsy?

Answer: Jewish law sanctions the performance of a post-mortem examination *only* where specific questions may be answered to enable immediate modification in the care of patients.

Comment: The subject of autopsy in Jewish law is an extremely complex one and, therefore, in a brief communication such as this, only a few basic principles can be enunciated. Further details will be provided in future mailings, lectures, symposia, and other forums planned by the Society. For guidance in a specific case, the physician is urged to seek consultation with a competent rabbinic authority.

It is recognized that, in United States law, consent for autopsy must be obtained from the next of kin. It is further recognized that it is the usual expectation in nearly all hospitals that consent be sought, by the house officer or attending physician, for the performance of a post-mortem examination on every patient who dies in the hospital, irrespective of the cause of death or age of the patient. Jewish law does *not* accept this approach. The preservation of the dignity of the deceased interdicts and prohibits autopsy solely for the purpose of establishing the cause of death, or to increase medical knowledge in general. Man was created in the image of God and may, therefore, not be desecrated in any way, except in circumstances such as illustrated below. Just as an observant Jewish physician refrains from doing certain prohibited acts on the Sabbath, so too must he refrain from participating in autopsy permission requests, except where Jewish law allows it.

Autopsy in Jewish law is permitted only to answer a specific question. The knowledge gained would then contribute to the immediate improved care of patients. For example, autopsy would be allowed where a patient received experimental chemotherapy for a neoplastic disease and the patient died, or where a patient received an experimental antibiotic or an untested vaccine for the treatment or prophylaxis of an infectious disease and the patient died, or where a patient underwent an operation in which a new or experimental surgical technique was employed and the patient died. In each of these situations, it is imperative to ascertain whether or not the drug or vaccine or surgical technique contributed to the patient's death. In addition, the effectiveness, or lack thereof, of the experimental drug, vaccine, or operation may be determined. Such information concerning the possible toxicities and/or benefits to the now deceased patient are critical in the physician's decision-making process regarding the possible use of the same drug, vaccine, or operation on other living patients.

There may also arise a rare instance where the patient dies of a genetic disorder or an infectious disease and an autopsy might answer a question (e.g., the etiologic agent may be found) that would have immediate relevance for genetic counselling, or for urgent prophylactic treatment of close contacts to the patient, respectively. This autopsy approval is based on the assumption that all antemortem tests were inconclusive, and that the information to be gained by performing an autopsy will indeed have immediate application to the living. In the case of an infection, there must be clear and firm presumptive evidence that the infectious agent possibly involved in the demise of the patient is one where immediate prophylaxis would be available, indicated, and effective. A patient who dies with fever and vague signs suggestive of an infection is *not* included in the above category; nor is a patient who dies of a suspected infection that can be determined at autopsy (e.g., cytomegalus virus infection) but where no effective prophylactic therapy exists. Medical researchers on Alzheimer's disease often request brain autopsies. If the patient was in an experimental therapeutic protocol, such a request might be valid. Routine examination of all brains of Alzheimer's disease patients in the hope of finding clues cannot be sanctioned in *halachah*. The motivation of the physician requesting the autopsy must be closely scrutinized so that the true clinical-pathological picture not be distorted.

Where an autopsy is permissible in Jewish law, the manner in which it is conducted is of crucial importance. The post-mortem examination must be a directed procedure to answer a specific question or questions. Therefore, the autopsy must be limited to those areas necessary to obtain the answers to the questions posed. Where post-mortem needle biopsies or peritoneoscopes can provide the information sought, an open procedure should not be condoned.

The autopsy itself should be done as a surgical procedure with the same dignity, respect, and consideration that would be accorded a living patient undergoing an operation. The autopsy should be performed in dignified surroundings. The deceased should be draped and only the area of incision exposed. Proper decorum should be observed, and the behavior of the surgical-pathological staff should be appropriate to the situation. Organs should *not* be removed from the body but examined in situ, except where the information needed cannot be obtained save by removing the organ or organs in question. Even then, *all* organs must be returned to the body for burial, except for small sections necessary for microscopic examination and for pathology "blocks" as required by law.

Ideally, the post-mortem examination should be performed in the presence of an observant Jewish physician, or clergyman, or some other reliable person to ensure that the aforementioned requirements are strictly adhered to. If this is not possible, then an autopsy permission form, specifying the above conditions, can be employed. This form would legally bind the hospital and pathology staff to perform the autopsy in the manner requested and signed for by the next of kin.

Subject: *Embalming.*

Question: Is the embalming of a body permissible in Jewish law?

Answer: Embalming is ordinarily prohibited in Jewish law.

Comment: As presently performed, embalming involves the following halachic problems:

1) The incisions over the major arteries where the embalming fluid is injected constitute a *nivul hamet* (desecration of the dead).

2) By injection of embalming fluid, the blood from the body is forced out from the major blood vessels; the blood is considered part of the body and requires burial.

3) Some embalmers either remove organs or aspirate and macerate organs as part of the embalming procedure. These acts are prohibited as *nivul hamet*.

4) Some embalmers inject a colored dye, or trim the nose or puff out the cheeks or perform other procedures for "cosmetic" reasons. All these acts are prohibited as *nivul hamet*.

If the body must be transported over great distances for burial (such as from the United States to Israel) and preservation of the body is desired (or required by law), it might be permissible to inject embalming fluid directly into major vessels or body cavities but *without* making any incisions and *without* performing any prohibited act such as illustrated in items 3 and 4 above. Any extruded blood should accompany the body for burial. Specific rabbinic approval must be obtained for each case.

Subject: *Burial of a fetus.*

Question: Does an unborn fetus require burial? If a woman spontaneously aborts a fetus, or if a therapeutic abortion is performed, does the fetus require burial?

Answer: An unborn fetus more than forty days old should be buried, if possible.

Comment: Until forty days after conception, an abortus does not require burial. After that time, however, attempts should be made to obtain the aborted fetus in order to effect burial. Although there is no absolute halachic requirement to bury a fetus, on moral grounds one should attempt to procure the fetus for burial, based on the tenet that man (including a fetus) was created in the image of God.

The distinction between before and after forty days with regard to burial in no way diminishes the right to life of a pre-forty-day fetus. A woman during the first forty days of gestation may not be aborted except for a threat to the mother's life or health. This right to life is further emphasized by the halachic permissibility and requirement to set aside all Sabbath laws to save the life of a fetus less than forty days old.

Pathological examination of the fetus prior to burial can be approved if there is information to be obtained that would help in future pregnancies.

Subject: *Burial of organs removed at surgery.*

Question: Do organs excised at surgery (e.g., gallbladder, stomach, prostate, uterus, etc.) require burial? Do amputated fingers, toes, or limbs require burial?

Answer: Excised organs *do not* require burial but amputated limbs *do* require burial.

Comment: Jewish law requires the burial of any organ or limb containing "flesh, sinews, and bones" (*basar, gidim, ve'atzamot*). Hence, internal soft tissue organs containing no bones, such as the appendix, stomach, gallbladder, lung, kidney, uterus, prostate, and intestine, do not require burial. However, a limb or finger or toe *does* require burial, since it fulfills the above criteria.

The aforementioned applies only to the surgical excision of an organ or limb from a live person. *Any* part of a dead body, whether or not it contains "flesh, sinews, and bones," *does* require burial, since it imparts ritual defilement.

HAZARDOUS THERAPY AND

HUMAN EXPERIMENTATION

Subject: *Bone marrow donation for transplantation.*

Question: Is a healthy person allowed or obligated to donate bone marrow for transplantation into another person (often a close relative) in an attempt to save the latter's life? Is the donor permitted or required to undergo the risk of the anesthesia and the discomfort of the multiple marrow punctures that are part of the procedure?

Answer and Comment: Since Judaism considers human life to be of infinite value, we are required to make every effort to save human life and to restore the sick to good health. Maimonides (Commentary to Nedarim 4:4) and others state that the scriptural phrase *and thou shalt restore it to him* (Deut. 22:2), which refers to the restoration of lost property, also includes the restoration of the health of one's fellow man, if he has lost it. Furthermore, the biblical admonition *neither shalt thou stand idly by the blood of thy neighbor* (Lev. 19:16) includes not only the obligation to save someone who is drowning or being mauled by beasts or attacked by robbers (Sanhedrin 73a) but also the obligation to save human life by healing the sick (Maimonides, *Hilchot Rotze'ach* 1:14). If there is no self-endangerment in the saving of human lives it is thus a biblical mandate to do so. However, when there is a measure of risk involved but it is not deemed to be excessive, the obligation is viewed by *halachah* as a voluntary one.

In the case of a bone marrow transplant, the risk and discomfort to the donor are sufficiently small compared with the near certainty of death for the recipient (who has presumably already received all other standard therapy) to permit bone marrow donation for transplantation. This situation is a classic example of the risk/benefit ratio where a small risk to one person's life may be undertaken to restore the health and save the life of a dangerously ill patient (*pikuach nefesh*). The donor, however, cannot be coerced into donating his bone marrow against his will. In the absence of voluntary informed consent, no one may halachically be subjected to so invasive a procedure even if the procedure may be life-saving. Thus, incompetent or retarded adults or children cannot serve as donors.

Subject: *Donation of cadaver organs for transplantation.*

Question: May a person will his organs for transplantation? Must a specific recipient be at hand? May one donate one's corneas to a cornea bank?

Answer: The donation of specific organs from a cadaver, where death has been determined by halachic criteria, is not in violation of any halachic ruling.

Comment: The overriding consideration of saving a life (*pikuach nefesh*) sets aside all biblical laws including the prohibitions of mutilation of the dead, deriving benefit from the dead, and delaying the burial of the dead. Hence to donate one's kidneys to save another's life is certainly permissible.

A blind person is considered by most rabbinic opinion to be in the category of the dangerously ill (*choleh sheyesh bo sakana*) and those for whom the principle of *pikuach nefesh* would apply. Hence corneal transplants are also permissible.

Heart transplants are now considered therapeutic and not experimental and are therefore halachically acceptable if the death of the donor has been halachically established and the risk/benefit ratio to the recipient meets halachic standards.

The voluntary donation removes all questions of dishonoring the dead and sets aside any concern for deriving benefit from the dead. It is also allowed to donate one's corneas to an eye bank without having a specific recipient in mind, since it is most probable the cornea will be used immediately. Hence the recipient is considered to be "at hand" (*lefanenu*).

Subject: *Donation of organs and blood from live donors.*

Question: Is a person allowed to subject himself to the danger, however small, of an operative procedure to remove one of his kidneys in order to save the life of another? May one donate a pint of blood to a blood bank?

Answer: A living person may donate a kidney to save another's life. It is also permissible to donate blood to a blood bank.

Comment: In a previous answer, we discussed the donation of cadaver organs for transplantation. Concerning the use of a living donor, the question arises as to the possible transgression of the biblical commandments *Take heed to thyself and keep thy soul diligently* (Deut. 4:9) and *Take ye therefore good heed unto yourselves* (Deut. 4:15). The Talmud (Berachot 32b) and Maimonides (*Hilchot Rotzeach* 11:4) interpret these verses to be biblical prohibitions against subjecting oneself to any physical danger, since it is not permitted to intentionally wound oneself (Baba Kamma 91b and Codes); and one may not forfeit a life to save another (Oholot 7:6 and Codes); can one therefore endanger one's life by donating a kidney in order to save another's life?

The answer, based on the Babylonian Talmud and adopted by most of the codes of Jewish law, is that one is allowed (or obligated, according to some authorities) to place oneself into a possibly dangerous situation to save his fellow from certain death. The donor *endangers* his life to save the recipient from *certain* death. Hence, a donor may endanger his own life or health to supply an organ to a recipient whose life would thereby be saved, provided the probability of saving the recipient's life is substantially greater than the risk to the donor's life or health.

Giving a pint of blood is akin to an organ donation. It is permissible to give blood to a blood bank even without a specific recipient in mind because there is a reasonable certainty of the blood being used. The danger to the donor is minimal while the benefit to the recipient may be life-saving.

Sources: Shulchan Aruch, Orach Chayim 330:8 and Choshen Mishpat 426. See commentary Pitchei Teshuvah on the latter.

Subject: *Hazardous surgery and human experimentation.*

Question: Is a patient allowed to accept and/or is the physician permitted to perform hazardous surgery? Is an experimental treatment with a new drug or vaccine permissible? Under what circumstances?

Answer and Comment: Jewish law is categorically opposed to any form of experimentation in which the human organism serves as an experimental animal, if there is the slightest hazard to the individual taking part in the experiment, without concomitant benefit to the *same* individual. Even the informed voluntary consent of an individual does not suffice to permit the physician to subject him to possibly hazardous medical procedures.

The evaluation of new surgical procedures, or the multiphasic study of new pharmacological agents, can occur only within a therapeutic protocol. If a patient is suffering from an illness for which there is no known medical treatment, he may then be subjected to new procedures if there is valid expectation of benefiting this patient. A careful evaluation of experiments done on animals should enable the physician to review the expected beneficial results, as well as the potential hazards of a new medical procedure. Only if the expectation of beneficial results exceeds the danger of causing harm to the patient can this new treatment be instituted.

Whenever the physician cannot recommend, on the basis of sound scientific principles, a specific experimental procedure, he is forbidden to offer it as "one chance in a million." It is a fundamental tenet of our faith that the personal God does not permit a patient to be "left to chance." The physician acts under a license restricted to actions definable on the basis of scientific principles, and must restrict himself to such actions.

When specific treatment cannot be recommended because of inadequate information as to the potential hazards, then such treatment is forbidden in Jewish law.

Subject: *Hazardous surgery.*

Question: Is it permissible to perform dangerous surgery that may hasten death in a patient who cannot survive long without surgical intervention?

Answer and Comment: In the situation where an operation may be dangerous but has a chance, albeit small, of healing the patient, if the patient will definitely die in a short time without the operation, it is permissible to proceed with the surgery. The major consideration in this matter is whether or not we have to be concerned about the short period of life or "life of the hour" (*chayey sha'ah*) that the patient would live without the surgery. This short time period may be sacrificed even if the surgery is unsuccessful and the patient's death is thereby hastened.

The Talmud (Abodah Zarah 27b) states that in a case where it is doubtful whether the patient will live or die, we must not let heathen physicians heal him (lest the heathen physicians intentionally aggravate the patient's condition or even kill him); but if the patient will certainly die, we may allow them to heal because we are not concerned with the short period of life the patient is expected to live (since there is the small chance that they may cure him). This position is codified in the Code of Jacob ben Asher (*Tur, Yoreh Deah* 155). The Talmud's position is also supported by the case of the four lepers (II Kings 7:4) who surrendered to the enemy and risked being killed rather than face certain death from starvation.

Therefore, if a patient will definitely die in a brief time period, we permit surgery to be undertaken even if the chance of success is remote and even if the surgery is unsuccessful the patient may die sooner. We are not concerned about the "life of the hour" since the surgery is for the patient's benefit because he may thereby be healed and live normally.

The risk/benefit ratio must be carefully weighed in each case. A 90 percent risk would be acceptable only if there is a 10 percent possibility of "healing the patient" (i.e., producing remission or cure). If palliation or minimal prolongation of life is the best one can expect, then such risks might not be halachically permissible.

Consultation with competent rabbinic authority is essential in all such cases.

Reference: Feinstein, M. *Iggrot Moshe. Yoreh Deah*, Part 2, 58, New York, 1973, pp. 77–78.

Subject: *Experimental instrumentation and phase I studies.*

Question: When is it permissible to use an experimental automatic defibrillator-pacemaker on humans? What restrictions, if any, are attendant upon its use?

Answer: If the following three areas of ethical-halachic concern have been satisfied, it would be permissible to use the experimental apparatus on humans: adequacy of animal experimentation to warrant a scale-up to human trials; informed consent of the patients; selection of patients who may personally benefit from the use of the apparatus so as not to merely evaluate a new technology solely for the benefit of others.

Comment: To use any new experimental device or drug on humans requires adequate evidence of the safety and efficacy of the instrument. Even the use of standard procedures in surgery, or pharmaceuticals in internal medicine, involves a "probability judgment" that makes every patient a "new experiment." If in the physician's considered judgment the level of doubt about the safety and efficacy of the new procedure has been reduced to that accompanying other medical protocols, then the move from animals to humans *is* warranted.

Since the first patients will be those undergoing open-heart surgery, some defibrillator-pacemaker device is needed as part of the surgical protocol. The substitution of the experimental instrument for the standard one has the possibility of offering specific benefit to the patient by virtue of the lower voltages required and the increased safety during postoperative monitoring that an automatic defibrillator-pacemaker offers. The potential adverse reaction seems to be limited to thermal injury at the electrodes' contact points—an injury that carries no foreseeable fatal consequence.

The same principles apply to the use of experimental chemotherapy, immunotherapy, or other experimental procedures on human subjects.

The patient surely has the right to demand standard practice. If, however, he can clearly understand the details of the procedural modifications and gives his *uncoerced consent*, there is no ethical or moral objection to beginning such clinical trials.

Subject: *Experiments on organs removed at surgery.*

Question: Is it permitted to perform experiments upon organs removed at surgery?

Answer and Comment: The prohibition of deriving benefit from the dead is not applicable to an organ removed from a live person. There is a question, however, as to whether or not an organ or flesh from a living person requires burial either because the law (*halachah*) requires burial (see Nazir, fol. 43) or because burial would avoid the possibility of a priest becoming ritually defiled by touching such an organ. If the organ or flesh is less than an olive's bulk in size (i.e., very small), it certainly does not require burial.

It seems more logical, however, that the question of burial relates only to preventing the organ or flesh from being treated with disrespect. This goal can be accomplished by burning or otherwise destroying the flesh or organ. R. Yose (Oholot 4:2) asserts that even an organ from a dead body can be burned (and does not require burial); certainly his ruling would apply to an organ removed at surgery from a living person.

Therefore, it is permissible to perform experiments on organs removed at surgery provided one buries or burns or otherwise destroys the remnants thereof at the conclusion of the experiment, without allowing the organ to be treated with disrespect.

Reference: Feinstein, M. *Iggrot Moshe, Yoreh Deah,* Responsum 232, New York, 1959, pp. 483–484.

Subject: *Animal experimentation.*

Question: Is a physician or scientist allowed to perform experiments on animals to obtain knowledge that can be used in the healing of the sick? Are there any restrictions?

Answer: Animal experimentation is permitted in Jewish law.

Comment: Jewish law sanctions medical research on animals, including vivisection. Unlike our fellow human beings, animals are in man's service. However, it is a violation of biblical law to cause unnecessary pain or suffering to animals, and such acts are prohibited as cruelty against animals. During medical research experiments, every precaution must be taken to protect the animal from unnecessary suffering or discomfort. Experiments designed to promote human health are in keeping with the religious rules governing man's relation with infrahuman species. The above regulations apply to all animals, large or small, primate, reptile, rodent, or otherwise.

MENTAL HEALTH

Subject: *Assertiveness against one's parents during psychotherapy.*

Question: If a psychiatrist recommends that a patient show assertiveness against his parents to help cure his emotional or mental illness, can the patient do so? Does the biblical commandment *Honor thy Father and thy Mother* (Exod. 20:12 and Deut. 5:16) prohibit such assertiveness?

Answer: Assertiveness against one's parents in certain circumstances (described below) is permissible. Aggression and disobedience are prohibited.

Comment: The commandment *Honor thy Father and thy Mother* is described in detail in the Code of Jewish Law (*Shulchan Aruch* 240:1–25). Unquestioning obedience is not synonymous with honor and respect. Jewish law (*halachah*) does not forbid opposition to or disagreement with parents but requires that such disagreement be expressed with honor and respect. This concept is exemplified in the *Shulchan Aruch* (*Yoreh Deah* 240:11):

> If one observes his father violating a Torah precept, he should not admonish him by saying, "You have transgressed a Torah precept"; rather he should point out to him: "Father, it is written in the Torah thus and thus" as if he is asking his father a question but not as if he is admonishing him so that his father will understand by himself and not be embarrassed.

Within the commandment *Honor thy Father and thy Mother* is included the obligation of caring for the physical and emotional needs of one's parents. Thus, if one's parents are senile or emotionally or mentally disturbed, one must still care for them to the best of one's ability (*Yoreh Deah* 240:10). Even if a parent is in gross violation of proper behavior toward a child, e.g., throws a precious object of the child into the ocean (*Yoreh Deah* 240:8), the child must remain silent and not publicly embarrass the parent. Any objections must be made in private or through formal procedures as by intervention of a competent rabbi. Such procedures, including the summoning of one's father into court over a financial dispute, are discussed by the glossary of R. Moses Isserles (*Rama*) in *Shulchan Aruch* (*Yoreh Deah* 240:8).

Halachah prohibits a parent from "leaning heavily" on his

children in *demanding* respect and obedience (*Yoreh Deah* 240:19) concerning minor matters. *Halachah* specifically exempts a child from listening to a parent who objects to the choice of a marriage partner or to the choice of school for Torah study even if it be in a distant land (*Yoreh Deah* 240:25). A father who has a dispute with another family cannot prohibit his child from having social contact with that family (*Yoreh Deah* 240:16).

In addition to the honor and respect due one's parents under the commandment *Honor thy Father and thy Mother,* one is also obligated to show gratitude to one who has rendered services or has done favors on one's behalf (*hakoras tov*), whether it was a parent or a stranger. The parents, as providers of all the needs of a child, are entitled to the thanks and gratitude of the recipient. Thus, the requirement to extend courtesies and honor and respect to one's parents, including good manners, expressions of concern and interest, and care for their good and welfare stems from two sources:

1) parental prerogatives under the commandment *Honor thy Father and thy Mother.*

2) the fundamental ethical principle of the Torah of showing gratitude to one who has done you favors.

Assertiveness against one's parents is not equivalent to aggression or disobedience; the latter two are forbidden in relation to one's parents. If assertiveness is recommended as part of a psychotherapeutic regimen, it has halachic approval if due courtesy, respect, tone of voice, and proper choice of language toward one's parent are maintained. If assertiveness is merely the first step in rebellion against parental authority and Torah life-style—and thus represents psychiatric sanction to accede to anti-halachic tendencies in stepwise fashion: assertiveness, aggressiveness, rebellion against religious teachings of home and community—it is clearly prohibited. The psychiatrist would then be imposing his own value system (which may be an immoral intrusion into the privacy of his patient with overtones of thought control) when he criticizes the life-style of the patient's family by suggesting violation of parental standards and life-style. If the tensions induced by specific traditional modes of conduct (e.g. chassidic garb, involvement with a "rebbe") are interfering with the psychotherapeutic process, careful consultation with a rabbi trained in this area is critically necessary.

Subject: *Treatment of mental illness by irreligious psychiatrists.*

Question: May psychiatrists who are irreligious (*minim*) or agnostic (*kofrim*) treat mental illness?

Answer and Comment: The question is whether or not patients with emotional or mental illness who need treatment from psychologists or psychiatrists are permitted to seek therapy from irreligious or agnostic practitioners. One should *not* go to such therapists because the therapies usually involve only words. The patient is healed by relating his thoughts to the therapist who then advises the patient how to conduct himself. One must certainly be concerned that the therapist may give advice contrary to the laws of the Torah and even contrary to the fundamental tenets of our faith and contrary to the proper practice of continence and modesty.

One cannot compare the healing that patients with other illnesses seek from irreligious and agnostic practitioners because the various types of medications with which they heal have no relationship to their agnosticism. The prohibition of obtaining healing from agnostic physicians applies only to therapies and incantations as cited in Abodah Zarah fol. 27 (*vide Tosafot*) and in the *Shulchan Aruch* (*Yoreh Deah* 155).

However, one must certainly be concerned that psychologists and psychiatrists whose entire therapy consists of verbal analyses and analytical deductions may speak words of agnosticism and profanity or impose their value system on their patients. But if they are expert physicians and promise that they will not speak words that are contrary to the tenets of our faith or the commandments of the Torah, one might be able to rely upon them because experts do not lie. Therefore, one should certainly try to locate a psychiatrist who is an observant Jew. If none is available, one should arrange with the therapist that he not speak on matters relating to the Jewish faith or the religious life-style.

Reference: Feinstein, M. *Iggrot Moshe, Yoreh Deah*, Part 2, 57, New York, 1973, p. 77.

Subject: *Mood modifying drugs.*

Question: Are there any restrictions on the physician in prescribing psychotropic or psychopharmacological medications such as antipsychotics, antidepressants, anxiolytics, and long-term agents such as lithium and disulfiram?

Answer: Psychotropic drugs are useful in the total care of the patient when anxiety or depression is of such an intensity as to be incapacitating and, hence, the physician is medically and halachically justified in prescribing them for such a patient.

However, the indiscriminate use of such drugs without medical supervision should be discouraged. The possibility of addiction, with its impact on man's independence, is especially abhorrent, unless a competent medical authority judges that such addiction is necessary to control intractable pain.

Comment: The physician prescribing psychotropic medications has the same obligations as any physician concerning the possible untoward complications of medication and the overall risk benefit ratio. It is possible for patients to misuse medication and to worsen the condition for which the medication was originally intended. So too, patients in certain categories of psychiatric illness can request psychotropics long after the time when it is possible for them to deal with their difficulties without medication. The danger of drug dependence, physiological or psychological, is of course a particular concern when psychotropic medications are prescribed and is among the most serious side effects of their usage. Since the physiologically addictive states consequent to drug misuse are of considerable variety, the physician is obligated to be knowledgeable about this danger and take all necessary precautions to foresee the dangers in prescribing medications with such a potential. The decision as to when and when not to treat psychiatric symptoms pharmacologically is a medical decision dependent on current recognized standards of psychopharmacotherapeutic drug use, as well as the physician's own clinical judgment.

The use of the psychotropic drugs on the Sabbath poses specific questions in terms of health needs. Will the omission of a routine dose of a psychotropic medication have negative health effects or impede recuperation? It can be argued that where relief of severe anxiety or tension is the major goal of the medication prescribed, the sabbatical ban on the use of medication should not be applied. In addition, the maintenance medications are dependent on a sustained blood level of active drug for their therapeutic value, and interrupting the regular use would clearly disrupt the treatment course and effect. For example, lithium maintenance therapy would become highly unpredictable if subject to regular lapses in use.

Similarly, the use of antipsychotics, e.g., haloperidol or perphenazine, and antidepressants, e.g., imipramine or amitryptiline, during *acute* phases of psychiatric disorders would be seriously handicapped by interruptions in the prescribed course. During the acute phase of schizophrenic or depressive psychoses the rapid control of symptoms is a vital goal of psychopharmacological treatment and should have no interruptions.

Subject: *Sex change in adults.*

Question: Is an adult Jew (male or female) allowed to undergo a medical and/or surgical sex change?

Answer: Jewish law prohibits sex change operations.

Comment: Surgical procedures or medical intervention (i.e., hormonal therapy) to effect a sex change in an adult is strictly forbidden for a variety of reasons, including the prohibitions of castration (*sirus*) and homosexuality (*mishkav zachar*).

Surgery not recognized as necessary for correction of anatomic or physiological abnormalities is viewed as an act of mutilation. The psychological stresses that underlie the patient's request for such self-mutilation must be dealt with by psychiatric therapy, not surgery.

If in violation of Torah law such a sex change operation was performed, the individual maintains his presurgical sex with all its halachic implications.

DENTISTRY

Subject: *Dental prostheses, fillings, and bridges, and ritual immersion (tevilah).*

Question: Is a temporary or permanent dental prosthesis, filling, or bridge considered an impediment to the proper performance of *tevilah*? Do any of the above constitute an impediment or barrier (*chatzitzah*) between the person and the water? Must such prostheses be removed before *tevilah*?

Answer: Dental fillings and all permanent dental prostheses are *not* a *chatzitzah*; *tevilah* is permitted without their removal.

Comment: All permanent bridgework, or cemented or wired (i.e., permanent) braces do *not* constitute an interposing barrier (*chatzitzah*) and therefore do *not* hinder the regular process of *tevilah*. However, removable dentures, removable braces, removable bridges, and the like *must* be removed before *tevilah*.

All fillings, whether temporary or permanent, that were fashioned by a skilled dentist are not a *chatzitzah*. *Tevilah* may be performed without their removal *unless* they have been improperly placed and must be removed and corrected by the dentist. *Tevilah* must be postponed until such correction is made. For example, a filling that is interfering with chewing and must be corrected by the dentist, or a bridge that is painful because further correction must be made on the device, should be fixed before *tevilah*.

The application of a surgical dressing to the gums during extensive gum work may require a delay in the time of *tevilah*. Rabbinic consultation should be sought in such cases as each case must be decided upon by the particular circumstances of that case.

An orthodox Jewish dentist should advise his patient that a particular dental procedure may involve halachic problems concerning *tevilah*. In such instances he should recommend rabbinic consultation.

Subject: *Separate dentures for Passover.*

Question: Must a patient with false dentures secure a separate set for the Passover holiday? Are separate dentures for *milchig* ("milk") and *fleishig* ("meat") required all year round?

Answer: Separate dentures are *not* required for Passover or for *milchig* and *fleishig*.

Comment: Since food that is eaten does not usually reach a degree of temperature that surpasses the pain threshold, approximately 50°C or 120°F (*yad soledet bo*), no absorption of food by the teeth is considered to occur. Therefore, separate dentures for "meat" and "milk" foods are not required.

It is recommended, however, that someone with false dentures should not chew hard *chametz* on the day before Passover eve because of a legal technicality based upon the rabbinical consideration called *ducheka desakina*, i.e., effect of pressure in causing absorption. Because of the unusual severity of Passover law, the false denture user is advised not to chew hard *chametz* from noon of the day before Passover eve onward. He does *not*, however, have to procure a separate set of dentures for the Passover holiday.

If dentures or bridges are removable, they should be soaked for a twenty-four-hour period prior to the holiday after careful brushing to remove all particulate matter.

Dental Emergencies on the Sabbath*

Introduction

It is axiomatic in Judaism that human life is of infinite value. The preservation of human life takes precedence over all biblical commandments and rabbinic enactments except three: idolatry, murder, and incest.[1] In order to preserve human life, all ritual laws, save the above three, are suspended for the overriding consideration of saving a human life.[2]

How does the practicing dentist apply this basic principle when confronted with an emergency or potential emergency on the Sabbath? What constitutes a dental emergency requiring the dentist to set aside all Sabbath laws to treat his patient? Under what circumstances may the dentist open his office on the Sabbath, turn on the lights, prepare and apply medications, cements, fillings, and their like, use the drill, incise an oral abscess, and perform other therapeutic procedures for his suffering patient?

Abrogation (Hutra) or Suspension (Dechuya) of the Sabbath

One of the most renowned halachic controversies concerning medical care on the Sabbath is the question whether danger to life (*pikuach nefesh*) or potential danger to life completely sets aside the biblical laws and rabbinic rules and regulations pertaining to the Sabbath (*hutra*), or whether this danger only suspends them (*dechuya*). This famous controversy of whether the Sabbath is *hutra* or *dechuya* for *pikuach nefesh* is more theoretical than practical. Theoretically, if the Sabbath is *hutra*, it is as if the Sabbath does not exist and, therefore, the Jewish dentist may act in accord with standard dental procedures in treating his patient with *pikuach nefesh* on the Sabbath similar to that which he would do on a weekday for that patient. (Of course, even if the Sabbath is consid-

*Reprinted with permission from the *Journal of Halacha and Contemporary Society* #14, Fall 1987 (Sukkot 5748), pp. 49–64.

ered *hutra*, this would apply only to care of the *patient;* it does not mean, for example, that the dentist could do other work just because he is taking care of a critically ill person.) If the Sabbath, however, is only *dechuya*—suspended or set aside only for the *pikuach nefesh* situation—the dentist would have to limit himself to those dental procedures absolutely essential to take care of the dental emergency.

However, it is clear from the codes of Jewish law, including the *Shulchan Aruch*[3] and *Mishneh Torah*,[4] that a physician or dentist must perform all acts required for the care of his patient (*kol tzorchei choleh*) and not limit himself exclusively to those things which would remove the danger to life (*pikuach nefesh*).[5] The medical or dental practitioner must do everything that he would ordinarily do for his patient on a weekday. Thus, from a practical standpoint, this major distinction between *hutra* and *dechuya* is irrelevant once the patient's condition has been classified as *pikuach nefesh*.[6]

A second theoretical difference between *hutra* and *dechuya* is in the use of a non-Jewish dentist who is equally competent. If the Sabbath is *hutra* for *pikuach nefesh*, there is no need to send the patient to the non-Jewish dentist and the Jewish dentist himself can treat the patient on the Sabbath as if the Sabbath were nonexistent. If, however, the Sabbath is *dechuya*, or only temporarily suspended for *pikuach nefesh*, there is no need for the Jewish dentist to transgress the Sabbath and the patient can be cared for by the non-Jewish dentist. However, contrary to this line of reasoning, our Sages rule that even if the Sabbath is *dechuya* for *pikuach nefesh* situations, the most competent Jewish medical or dental practitioners and not a non-Jew should care for the patient. Maimonides[7] clearly states that "when such things have to be done [to save a life on the Sabbath] . . . they should not be left to heathens, minors, slaves, or women, but should be done by adult and scholarly Israelites." Thus, if an illness is classified as *pikuach nefesh*, it is not proper to refer the patient to a non-Jew. There is no distinction in this regard in practice between *hutra* and *dechuya*. The author of *Mishnah Berurah*[8] concurs that this is the accepted halachic practice.

A real distinction between *hutra* and *dechuya* might be the performance of an act on the Sabbath in an unusual manner (*shinuy*) thereby changing the offence from a biblical to a rabbinic transgression. If the Sabbath is *hutra* for *pikuach nefesh*, the dentist may perform all acts necessary to treat his patient in the same manner he would perform them on a weekday. If, however, the Sabbath is only temporarily set aside for *pikuach nefesh*, it would seem preferable to use a *shinuy* to perform all therapeutic acts on the Sabbath in order to lessen the transgression from a biblical to a rabbinic offense.

What is a *shinuy* for a dentist? If a right-handed dentist performs root canal work with his left hand, that might be considered a *shinuy*, but this is obviously highly impractical. The definition of *shinuy* requires that the act be performed in a less competent manner than usual so that either the results of the act are less good or the method is more difficult. Rav Abraham Borenstein, known as *Avnei Nezer*, in the introduction to his work *Egley Tal*, specifically states that a *shinuy* is when the outcome of an act is less successful or the method of doing the act is particularly tedious. If neither definition applies, it is not a *shinuy*. Turning the light on with one's elbow or starting the dental drill with one's knee is not a *shinuy*, according to Rav Moshe Feinstein,[9] because the *shinuy* of using one's elbow or knee is an act (turning on the light or starting the drill) that does not affect the electrical contact that sets into motion the forbidden activity. It is, therefore, usually not feasible for a dentist to employ a *shinuy* that is halachically valid in the direct care of his patient with *pikuach nefesh* on the Sabbath.

In practical terms for the dentist, therefore, there is no distinction between *hutra* and *dechuya*. Once a situation has been classified as *pikuach nefesh*, the Jewish dentist is obligated to do everything necessary to care for his patient on the Sabbath and that should be his only concern.

Definition of Pikuach Nefesh *(Danger to Life)*

A frequent halachic question in dentistry is whether or not the presence of an abscess is considered to be *pikuach nefesh* requiring incision and drainage on the Sabbath. The halachic definition of *pikuach nefesh* is not the same as the medical-dental definition of danger to life. *Halachah* sets a higher standard of risk/benefit, i.e., a lower level of risk or danger than set by medicine is classified as *pikuach nefesh* by the *halachah*. Thus, any internal sore from within the lips and mouth, including the teeth, is halachically considered to be a situation of *pikuach nefesh*,[11] if that sore might lead to an actual or potential danger to life. Our Sages were especially cognizant of the fact that any infection in the mouth is potentially dangerous because of the direct circulatory connections between the oral cavity and the brain. The fact that total asepsis in the mouth is nearly impossible to achieve is compensated by God's creation of protective enzymes, antibodies, and other host defense systems which protect the body from sepsis secondary to the bacterial flora of the oral cavity. The fact that any "significant" infection or inflammation or abscess in the mouth can today be treated prophylactically and/or therapeutically with antibiotics in no way eliminates the classification of that abscess or infection as *pikuach nefesh* requiring the dentist to treat it on the Sabbath. Thus, conditions such as tooth abscesses, jaw swellings, gum infections, and their like are all defined in the category of internal sore (*makah shel chalal*) for which Sabbath laws must be put aside in favor of the most effective and expeditious dental care.

A cancre sore or a broken orthodontist's wire or a mild tooth discomfort and their like are not considered to be *pikuach nefesh* although one could stretch the above reasoning *ad absurdum* and say that any scratch or pimple in the mouth could lead to infection, abscess formation, and brain infection. What is called *pikuach nefesh* must be "significant" pathology. Man is mortal and every human being is subject to an occasional scratch or pimple on his body. "All is by the hand of Heaven except colds and fevers"[12] means that every person can have an occasional cold and/or fever. The norm or baseline is not perfection. A cold or minor sore is not a pathological condition to be classified as *pikuach nefesh*. However, a well-established infection in the mouth is clearly a case of *pikuach nefesh*.

Categories of Illness Other Than Pikuach Nefesh

There are four classic halachic categories of illness in relation to the suspension of Sabbath laws: *pikuach nefesh* (danger or possible danger to life), *choleh she'ayn bo sakanah* (ill person but without danger to life), *meychush be'alma* (minor discomfort), and *chesron eyver* (chance of loss of function of an organ or limb). Elsewhere,[13] one of the authors of this essay provides an analysis which suggests that there is a fifth category—*choleh she'ayn bo sakanah im tzar gadol* (ill person without danger to life but with great pain or discomfort).[14] This category is tantamount to *chesron eyver* in that it is permissible for such a patient to waive all rabbinic prohibitions in addition to telling a non-Jew to do the act (amira le'akum).[15]

Pikuach nefesh has already been discussed in the previous section of this essay. Choleh she'ayn bo sakanah[16] refers to a patient who is suffering from an illness which does not constitute a danger to life or limb but is serious enough or painful enough to make the patient feel that he would rather be in bed (mutal lemishkav). A patient with a bad toothache due to an exposed nerve but without infection should be classified in this category. For such a patient to whom there is no danger to life, therapeutic intervention on the Sabbath may only set aside the rabbinic prohibition of telling a non-Jew to do the act (amira le'akum). The treatment should, therefore, be provided by a non-Jew.

Meychush be'alma refers to minor discomfort for which the taking of any medication is a rabbinic prohibition. Our Sages were concerned that because of discomfort, the person may overact (bohul al gufoh) and allow himself some unwarranted leniencies in Sabbath observances.

Chesron eyvor refers not to the loss of an organ or limb but to the loss of normal function of a limb.[17] This category of medical condition is halachically classified in between pikuach nefesh and choleh she'ayn bo sakanah. The Avnei Nezer exemplifies chesron eyver as an orthopedic problem such as a torn ligament or muscle which, if not repaired on the Sabbath, would result in the patient's walking with a limp. Chesron eyver does not require actual loss of the limb.

Loss of a Tooth as Chesron Eyver

Is a tooth in the category of chesron eyver for which a Jew can set aside all rabbinic prohibitions on the Sabbath? The third opinion in the Shulchan Aruch[18] concerning chesron eyver is the ruling we follow, namely, a Jew is allowed to waive rabbinic prohibitions in order to preserve a limb or its function. If a patient presents to the dentist on the Sabbath following trauma with two avulsed adult teeth, one could argue that halachah considers this situation as chesron eyver requiring the immediate reimplantation of those teeth. Teeth are not cited in the Mishnah in Oholot which lists the 248 eyvorin (limbs or organs) of the body. However, teeth can be halachically classified as *eyver* based on *Avnei Nezer's* definition of *chesron eyver* cited above. Less than the normal use of a limb is *chesron eyver*. Since the jaw is an *eyver* and the absence of teeth interferes with its proper functioning, and since the reimplantation of those teeth would restore the proper functioning of the jaw, the traumatic avulsion of teeth represents a situation of *chesron eyver*.

If this analysis is correct, it is permissible to reimplant an adult tooth on the Sabbath provided one does not violate any biblical (*d'oraitha*) prohibitions. A non-Jew is obviously very helpful in this situation because whatever he does for the Jewish dentist on the Sabbath is only rabbinic and not biblical in its implications. In the absence of a non-Jew, is the Jewish dentist permitted to drill, mix paste or cement, cut wires, apply wax, make dental impressions, turn on lights, etc., on the Sabbath in order to reimplant a traumatically avulsed tooth? Each of these activities must be evaluated as to whether it involves one or more biblical or rabbinic prohibitions.

A Practical Suggestion

Which activities in the sophisticated modern dentist's office would be classified as rabbinic prohibitions on the Sabbath which may be waived for the sake of *chesron eyver?* Turning on lights on the Sabbath, according to many rabbinic authorities, is a biblical offense. Mixing cement or paste is a biblical offense known as *lishah*. *Lishah* (kneading) is the mixing of water and fine particles to form a dough or paste. There is no *shinuy* possible with *lishah* since the end result is the same, i.e., the making of a paste or cement. Premade cements in tubes that can be squeezed out, if available, might be acceptable for Sabbath use. Another method is for two people to make the cement together employing the suggestion of *shenayim she'osu* (see below). Pushing wax into a crevice is a biblical offense known as *memachek* (smoothing or waxing). Cutting a wire with one's left hand if one is right-handed constitutes a *shinuy* but is not practical. Starting the dentist's drill by turning on the motor on the Sabbath may or may not constitute a biblical offense. Most authorities rule that if the motor has no heating element, starting it on the Sabbath would only be classified as a rabbinic prohibition and permissible for a situation of *chesron eyver*. Obviously, it is rather difficult for a dentist to function on the Sabbath by suspending only rabbinic but not biblical prohibitions.

A practical suggestion for dentists who must treat a patient with *chesron eyver* or *choleh she'ayn bo sakanah im tzar gadol* is the intriguing approach of two people performing a single act. *Shenayim she'osu* converts every prohibited act on the Sabbath into a rabbinic prohibition. Rambam clearly states[19] that whenever two persons jointly do work that can be done by each one of them alone, they are exempt, and it does not matter if each one does a different part of the work, or whether both do the work together from beginning to end. It is a functional practical solution.[20] *Shenayim she'osu* is like a *shinuy* and considered to be a technical avoidance of a biblical prohibition. If the dentist and an attendant or family member or other bystander simultaneously start the drill, only a rabbinic prohibition is involved, which is waived for *chesron eyver* on the Sabbath. Once the drill is running, the dentist can operate it alone until the procedure is completed.

Some authorities consider starting a dentist's drill to be a rabbinic prohibition if there is no heat or electricity involved in starting the motor, but only if it is an air compressor. However, according to some authorities, starting a motor involves the biblical transgression of converting a useless non-functioning machine into a functioning drill (*metaken manah*). Manipulating or cutting into gums and other soft tissue in reimplanting avulsed teeth is known as *mechatech basar be'alma* and is permitted.

Concerning rabbinic prohibitions (*issurei d'rabbanan*), we have been taught that the Rabbis did not enact prohibitions in the face of severe pain (*bemakom tza'ar lo gazru bo rabbanan*). These considerations, combined within the definition of *chesron eyver* cited above, may allow the dentist to function comfortably within *halachah* to restore the function of a tooth on the Sabbath. This is an often-overlooked category of illness on the Sabbath—no danger of life but great pain. For this category, a Jew may transgress rabbinic but not biblical prohibitions on the Sabbath as discussed above.[21]

Dental Abscesses

The Talmud[22] considers the piercing of an abscess with a pin to relieve the turgidity and pain and evacuate the pus on the Sabbath (*mapis mursa*) to be a rabbinic prohibition. However, the incision and drainage of an abscess and the insertion of a drain requires the expertise of a physician (*ma'aseh uman*) and is, therefore, classified as a biblical prohibition. Thus, the opening of an abscess to remove pus can be either a rabbinic or biblical offense if performed on the Sabbath, depending upon how it is done. In dentistry, an oral abscess is nearly always categorized in *halachah* as *pikuach nefesh* and, therefore, all therapeutic measures necessary to treat the abscess must be employed in the most expeditious manner possible.

Although medically the incision and drainage of a dental abscess can be postponed until after the Sabbath and the patient given antibiotics, the difference between the medical and halachic definition of *pikuach nefesh* is such that once the condition is categorized as *pikuach nefesh*, definitive treatment must be instituted promptly and not postponed because of the Sabbath.

Dental Anesthesia

The administration of an injection by a physician on the Sabbath might involve the biblical prohibition of "wounding" (*chavalah*) because the physician first aspirates before giving the injection to avoid injecting directly into a blood vessel. If blood is aspirated into the syringe, that would constitute an act of *chavalah*. However, for the dentist, giving an injection of a local anesthetic in the mouth is only a rabbinic act and, therefore, permissible for *chesron eyver* as defined earlier in this essay. In dentistry, injections are mainly for pain relief and even if they induce some gum bleeding, it is considered unintentional (*davar she'ayn miskaven*) and not in the category of *pesik reysho* (dialectic term for an absolutely unavoidable result of an act). Furthermore, the dentist has no need for that blood; on the contrary, he would prefer that the injection cause no bleeding at all. For all these reasons, the giving of an oral injection of a local anesthetic on the Sabbath by a dentist is considered to involve only a rabbinic prohibition.

Returning Home After A Dental Emergency

When a dentist has completed the treatment of a dental emergency on the Sabbath he should close his office but not turn off the lights. Shutting off the drill is permitted if otherwise a considerable financial loss might be incurred (hefsed mamon) and the dentist might be reluctant to treat another patient on the Sabbath in the future.

If a dentist is called to the hospital on the Sabbath for a dental emergency, the halachic rules of his returning home are the same as for a physician or emergency medical technician returning from a medical emergency. This subject has been described in detail elsewhere.[23, 24] A dentist should not drive his own car home from the scene of a dental emergency (office, hospital, etc.) but should take a taxi or have his car driven by a non-Jewish driver to minimize the Sabbath prohibitions involved.

Miscellaneous Dental-Halachic Issues

1. Dental prostheses, fillings, bridges, and tevilah (ritual immersion).

Dental fillings and all permanent (i.e., functional) dental prostheses are not an impediment or barrier (chatzitzah) between a person and the water of a ritual immersion bath (mikvah). Tevilah may be performed without their removal unless they have been improperly placed and must be removed and corrected by the dentist. Tevilah must be postponed until such correction is made. For example, a filling that is interfering with chewing and must be corrected by the dentist, or a bridge that is painful because further correction must be made on the device, must be fixed before tevilah.[25]

The terms temporary and permanent are often misinterpreted since the main halachic criteria relating to chatzitzah is whether or not the filling or prosthesis is functional. If a woman has a permanent filling which is too high and cannot chew on it because it bothers her and it hurts, she cannot go to mikvah until it is ground down. On the other hand, if she has a temporary cement filling which is fully functional, she is allowed to go to mikvah since it is classified as part of the body. If the filling is not functional, it is considered a chatzitzah whether made of gold, cement, or plastic. If it is functional, it is considered as part of the natural growth process of the tooth and is not a chatzitzah. Semi-permanent orthopedic dental devices are to be discouraged unless absolutely necessary because of the halachic problems concerning *tevilah* which they raise. Sutures do not hinder *tevilah* by their presence.[26] Plastic teeth and *tevilah* is discussed by Rav Feinstein.[27]

In summary, all permanent bridgework, or cemented or wired (i.e., permanent) braces do not constitute an interposing barrier (*chatzitzah*) and therefore do not hinder the regular process of *tevilah*. However, removable dentures, removable braces, removable bridges, and the like must be removed before *tevilah*. The application of a surgical dressing to the gums during extensive gum work may require a delay in the time of *tevilah*. Rabbinic consultation should be sought in such cases as each case must be adjudicated based upon the particular circumstances of that case.

2. Separate Dentures for Passover?

Separate dentures are not required for Passover for *milchig* ("milk foods") and *fleishig* ("meat foods"). Since food that is eaten does not usually reach a degree of temperature or heat that surpasses the pain threshold, no absorption of food by the teeth is considered to occur. Therefore, separate dentures for "meat" and "milk" foods are not required. It is recommended, however, that someone with false dentures should not chew hard *chametz* on the day before Passover eve because of a legal rabbinical technicality based upon the effect of pressure in causing absorption.[28] Because of the unusual severity of Passover law, the false-denture-user is advised not to chew hard *chametz* from noon of the day before Passover eve onward. He does not, however, have to procure a separate set of dentures for the Passover holiday. If dentures or bridges are removable, they should be soaked for a twenty-four hour period prior to the holiday after careful brushing to remove all particulate matter.[29]

3. Kohen (Priest) Studying Dentistry

Under the usual academic conditions, a *kohen* is not permitted to study dentistry. Because of the requirement in United States medical schools that students take anatomy and pathology courses, it is impossible for a *kohen* to attend medical or dental school. Even if the assumption is made that most, if not all, cadavers are non-Jewish, ritual defilement of a *kohen* still occurs upon contact (*maga*) or by carrying (*massa*) of any dead body. The halachic distinction between Jew and Gentile concerns ritual defilement on being present in the same room with a cadaver (tumat ohel).

The same objections expressed concerning medical school apply to dental school. The latter curriculum also includes anatomical dissection which is forbidden to a kohen, irrespective of whether the cadaver is Jewish or non-Jewish. If, however, the dental student can avoid actual dissection and attend only as an observer, and if his early dentistry training does not include a human skull with its dentition, then there may be dispensation for a kohen studying dentistry. This possible restricted permissibility rests upon the fact that in the present era we follow the lenient halachic ruling that a non-Jewish corpse does not convey ritual defilement to people in the same room who do not have direct contact with it. Unlike the physician, the dentist is not usually involved with dying patients, death certificates, the mortuary, etc., which pose seemingly insoluble problems to a physician who is a kohen.[30]

4. Training in Hospitals with Sabbath Obligations

Is a physician or dentist obligated to seek training or employment or attending physician status at a hospital where there is minimum or no conflict between hospital policy and Sabbath observance? The answer is that a physician or dentist must seek association with the most reputable and prestigious hospital possible to ensure excellent training and continuing education. Jewish law requires that the physician or dentist acquire maximum skill and competence to practice his chosen profession. Therefore, he should forego personal comfort and convenience of training in a hospital that is sympathetic to his religious needs in favor of a hospital that will provide him with the best possible training, provided that he is certain of this fortitude in maintaining all halachic requirements, despite the less favorable environment. However, if the superior training is to be acquired at the price of Sabbath desecration, even of rabbinic ordinances only, the physician or dentist must forego the educational advantages of the prestigious hospital.[31]

Conclusion

The classic Codes of Jewish Law rule that "for any internal sore (makah shel challal) that is from the lip or teeth inward, and the teeth themselves are included, one must desecrate the Sabbath." Thus, conditions such as tooth abscesses, jaw swelling, gum infections, and the like, are all classified in the category of "internal sore." In such cases, the Sabbath laws must be put aside in favor of the most effective and expeditious dental care. Oral surgery requiring postoperative care is certainly classified as a danger-to-life situation (*pikuach nefesh*) for which the Sabbath must be desecrated. However, if the patient suffering from a dental condition has only a mild discomfort without much associated pain, no Sabbath law may be desecrated. If there is danger of loss of function (*chesron eyver*), rabbinic but not biblical prohibitions may be transgressed. If there is moderate pain but no real danger, only the prohibition of telling a non-Jew to act (*amira le'akum*) is suspended. In cases of extreme pain, the same rules that govern *chesron eyver* apply. The dentist has all the obligations of a medical practitioner in cases classified as *pikuach nefesh*.

REFERENCES AND NOTES

1. Maimonides, M. (Rambam) *Mishneh Torah, Hilchot Yesodei Hatorah* 5:2.
2. *Ibid. Hilchot Shabbat* 2:1.
3. *Shulchan Aruch, Orach Chayim* 328:4.
4. *Mishneh Torah, Hilchot Shabbat* 2:1.
5. *Mishnah Berurah* 328:14 and the commentaries of *Biur Halacha* and *Be'er Hetev* there where the question is discussed as to whether or not the Sabbath should be desecrated for something whose omission would not constitute a danger to life. Authorities supporting both opposing viewpoints are cited.
6. Although Rambam (*Hilchot Shabbat* 2:1) rules that the Sabbath is only suspended (*dechuya*) and not completely set aside (*hutra*) if human life is in danger, he nevertheless clearly states that whatever a skilled physician considers necessary should be done for the patient on the Sabbath. Rabbis Joseph Karo (*Keseph Mishneh*), Nisson Girondi (Ran), and Solomon ben Adret (Rashba) are also of the opinion that the Sabbath is only suspended (*dechuya*) for danger to life. However, Rabbi Moshe Isserles (Rama) in his Responsa no. 76 states that the Sabbath is completely set aside (*hutra*) if human life is in danger.
7. *Mishneh Torah, Hilchot Shabbat,* 2:3.
8. *Mishnah Berurah* 328:37.
9. Personal communication.
10. *Mishneh Torah, Hilchot Shabbat* 2:5.
11. *Shulchan Aruch, Orach Chayim* 328.
12. *Ketubot* 30a.
13. Tendler, M.D. *Bet Yitzchak,* Yeshiva University Press, 1987.
14.   a) The Talmud (*Ketubot* 6b) states that he who pierces an abscess on the *Shabbat*—if in order to cause the pus to come out of it—is free from punishment (and it is permitted). See also the commentary of *Tosafot* there, s.v. *ve'im lehatzi* which states that the Talmud is certainly concerned with a patient in pain but where there is no danger to life; nevertheless, the Rabbis did not enact a preventive measure to prohibit rabbinic "work" on the *Shabbat* even if performed by a Jew. See also *Shabbat* 107a.

   b) The Talmud (*Ketubot* 60a) states that a man suffering from pain in the chest (literally: groaning) may suck (goat's) milk (directly from the goat) on the Sabbath (even though the release of milk from the animal's udder resembles the plucking of a plant from its root, or the "unloading" of a burden which is ordinarily forbidden on the Sabbath). What is the reason?—continues the Talmud—because sucking is an "unusual" method of "unloading" against which, where pain is involved, no preventive measure was enacted by the Rabbis (even though the Jewish patient himself sucks the milk and does not ask a non-Jew to secure the milk for him).

c) Shulchan Aruch, Orach Chayim, no. 328:28 also rules that it is permitted to pierce a boil on the Sabbath to express the pus therefrom. Mishnah Berurah no. 328:28 cites the opinion of Tosafot that the permissive ruling is due to the fact that where pain is involved, the Rabbis did not enact a preventive measure.

d) Shulchan Aruch, Orach Chayim no. 328:33 also rules that a person suffering from pain in the chest is permitted to suck milk directly from a goat on the Sabbath because where pain is involved, the Rabbis did not enact a preventive measure. The author of Mishnah Berurah (ibid.) cites the explanation of Rabbi Nisson Girondi (Ran) that "although the rule in regard to patients in whom there is no danger to life is to tell a non-Jew to perform the act, here [in the case of chest pain] it is different because the cure for the patient's ailment is that he suck [the milk] himself." This means that if there is pain and suffering and the relief thereof cannot be provided by an act of a non-Jew, it is permissible for the Jew to do it himself even if there is no danger to life (pikuach nefesh) of danger about the loss of function of an organ or limb (chesron eyver).

e) One should add that on the second day of Yom Tov it is permitted for a Jew(ess) to personally apply medication on his (her) eyes even though on the first day of Yom Tov this act can only be performed by a non-Jew. Similarly, for all other rabbinic rules, the Rabbis allowed such acts to be performed by Jews on the second day of Yom Tov (Shulchan Aruch, Orach Chayim 496:2).

15. Tosafot on Ketubot 60a and Shulchan Aruch, Orach Chayim 328:28.
16. Shulchan Aruch, loc. cit.
17. Responsa Avnei Nezer, introduction to Egley Tal.
18. Shulchan Aruch, loc. cit.
19. Mishneh Torah, Hilchot Shabbat 1:15.
20. R. Moshe Feinstein used this rationale in dealing with the problem faced by the Israeli army concerning the intermittent running of the tank air-conditioner on Shabbat.
21. See Note 14.
22. Ketubot 6b, Shabbat 3a and 107a.
23. Responsa Iggrot Moshe, Orach Chayim, Part 4, no. 80.
24. Rosner, F. and Wolfson, W. "Returning on the Sabbath from a life-saving mission." Journal of Halacha and Contemporary Society no. 9, Spring 1985, pp. 53–67.
25. Responsa Iggrot Moshe, Yoreh Deah no. 97.

26. *Ibid. Yoreh Deah*, Part 2, no. 87.
27. *Ibid.* no. 88.
28. Rabbi Aron Felder in *Oholei Yeshurun* [p. 82, parag. 33, note 200]. See also Responsa *Tzitz Eliezer*, 9:25.
29. Rosner, F. and Tendler, M.D. *Practical Medical Halachah*, New York, Feldheim, 1980, p. 86.
30. *Shulchan Aruch, Yoreh Deah* 369, 371, and 372:2 and the commentary *Dagul Mir'vavah* on 372:2.
31. Rosner and Tendler. *loc. cit.* p. 116.

THE SABBATH

Subject: *Carrying on the Sabbath.*

Question: Is a physician permitted to carry his instruments, drugs, or other necessities on the street (*reshut harabbim*) when going to see a patient on the Sabbath? Can the house officer carry his instruments between buildings of a hospital complex? What is the law concerning handkerchiefs and keys and the like?

Answer: For a dangerously ill patient, it *is* permitted to carry the essential medical instruments and supplies on the Sabbath.

Comment: Assuming that the hospital complex is enclosed by gates, walls of buildings, tunnels, or overpasses, it is permitted to carry between and within buildings without restriction. Where one needs to enter a public thoroughfare, the following ruling applies. Under ordinary circumstances carrying instruments or other medical supplies in the street on the Sabbath is an act prohibited by the Torah. However, for a dangerously ill patient (*pikuach nefesh*), it is permitted to transport through a public thoroughfare the instruments and material absolutely necessary for the patient's care. Such items include the stethoscope, X rays, keys to narcotics or medication closets, sphygmomanometers, and the like. Wherever possible, and where no delay in time or loss of efficiency would result, the carrying of these materials should be effected in an unusual manner (*shinuy*) in order to change the prohibition of carrying on the Sabbath from a biblical to a rabbinic violation. Hooking one's stethoscope to one's belt is an example of carrying in an unusual manner.

A house officer is urged to leave duplicate medical tools and supplies he might need in the hospital before the Sabbath so that he not be required to carry from his home on the Sabbath. The physician in private practice is strongly urged to hire a non-Jewish attendant for the Sabbath, wherever this is possible, to carry his instruments for him and perform other otherwise prohibited functions on the Sabbath for him. The use of a *shabbos goy* for ministering to *any* ill patient is permitted.

Handkerchiefs, house keys, and other nonmedical items may *not* be carried through a public thoroughfare (i.e., the street) on the Sabbath even in an unusual manner (*shinuy*).

Subject: *Writing on the Sabbath.*

Question: May one write on the Sabbath under any circumstances? If so, under what circumstances? Is one allowed or obligated to use one's left hand (*shinuy*), or use a typewriter or some alternative method of writing when information needs to be recorded?

Answer: Writing on the Sabbath is permitted only when absolutely essential to save life, and where no alternative exists.

Comment: Writing or typing on the Sabbath is a biblical prohibition. Whatever writing can be postponed until after the Sabbath without endangering the proper care of a critically ill patient must be so delayed. The practicing physician is urged, wherever possible, to hire a non-Jewish attendant to do whatever writing is essential and perform otherwise prohibited acts on the Sabbath (driving the car, etc.). For the house officer, a nurse, clerk, hired secretary, or any other non-Jewish person available in the hospital might be asked to write items that need to be recorded on the Sabbath by hospital regulations. These items would include routine histories, physical examinations, routine medication and treatment orders, laboratory requisition slips, progress notes, and the like.

Where the above alternatives are not possible, and where it is essential to the preservation of life (defined below) that the physician write, then he is permitted to do so. Wherever possible, and where no delay in time or loss of efficiency would result, writing should be done in an unusual manner (*shinuy*). Writing with the left hand, in a right-handed person, is considered an unusual manner and is preferable to the use of a typewriter. Other examples of *shinuy* are holding the writing instrument in an unusual way or writing at an unusual slant. However, if a delay in time or loss of efficiency engendered by writing with a *shinuy* might in any way interfere with the care of a critically ill patient, then writing in the usual manner without a *shinuy* is permitted.

What is considered essential to the *preservation of life?* Certain illustrative cases will serve as general guidelines. For example, recording the initial relevant history and physical findings of a critically ill patient (e.g., following a heart attack) admitted to the hospital on Friday night is permitted. However, *only* information that is of significant or perhaps essential value to another physician who may be called upon to assist or take over the care of the patient may be recorded. This ruling excludes the writing of social, personal, family, and past medical and surgical histories except where directly relevant to the patient's present illness. Also excluded is the recording of physical findings that do not bear directly on the patient's immediate problem. Other examples of writing permitted on the Sabbath (with the reservations noted above) are the recording of the progress of a woman in labor, vital signs of a postoperative patient, and drug allergies or sensitivities.

If the physician's signature is required to obtain needed drugs (e.g., narcotics) or services (e.g., oxygen) for a seriously or dangerously ill patient, then he may sign his name. Although this signature is only a legal requirement unrelated to actual patient care, it must be classified as a necessary act, if the nurse refuses to provide the essential drugs or services to the patient without it, and thus the signature is permitted.

One is *not* permitted to sign a death or birth certificate on the Sabbath, even with a *shinuy*, since there is no issue of preserving life.

Subject: *Use of elevators on the Sabbath.*

Question: May a physician use an elevator on the Sabbath? To ride one floor or only more than three floors? Is there a difference between automatic elevators requiring the passenger to push a button and elevators operated by an employee? Suppose the elevator operator is Jewish or his religion is unknown? If the physician routinely walks up two flights during the week and only rides for three or more flights, must he abide by this "self-imposed" rule on the Sabbath? Is the physician in practice seeing a patient at home any different from the house officer in the hospital with regard to the use of an elevator on the Sabbath? May one "ride" down on the elevator on the Sabbath?

Answer: A physician may use the elevator on the Sabbath when responding to a call that warrants his services on the Sabbath.

Comment: Within the hospital confines, any call to the house officer or attending physician must be viewed as a call for a dangerously ill patient (*pikuach nefesh*), and response by the physician should be in the most direct and efficient manner. Similarly, when responding on the Sabbath to the home of a patient who has been ill with a disease that Jewish law would classify as "dangerous to life" (i.e., *pikuach nefesh*), the same rule holds. If the physician is making a house call that is partly social to a patient who is not critically ill, then the use of the elevator is not allowed.

The availability of a staircase is a factor only if walking up the stairs will not require more time than waiting for the elevator. Certainly for the lower floors, this fact is empirically true, unless the elevator doors happen to be open when the physician arrives. Even if the time element could be equated, if running up the stairs would leave the physician panting (aside from the risk to his own health), it would interfere with his sensitivity in the use of the stethoscope and other instruments and general evaluation of the patient. Therefore, if *delay* or *loss of efficiency* would result from the physician using the stairs, he is obligated to use the elevator to visit his dangerously ill patient.

If the elevator is of the automatic type, then the physician may operate it himself. If the elevator is of the nonautomatic variety, then the religion of the elevator operator is irrelevant, since the latter has the same permissibility to help in the care of the patient by bringing the physician to the patient. Riding down is governed by the same halachic considerations as is riding up on the elevator.

If no other seriously ill patient is waiting for his services, the physician should walk down rather than use the elevator.

Subject: *Use of the telephone on the Sabbath.*

Question: May a physician use the telephone on the Sabbath? To receive and/or to make calls? To answer a page? In the hospital? At the patient's home? In the physician's office?

Answer: For a patient in whom there exists danger to life, the physician may receive and make telephone calls.

Comment: A house officer may answer *all* phone calls or paging messages, since most if not all of his hospitalized patients are in the category of being considered dangerously ill. Most, if not all, messages a house officer receives in the hospital relate to his patients. The house officer may make such calls as are required to care for his seriously ill patient. He should not, however, make calls for non-emergency needs. For example, he should not call the laboratory to obtain results of an elective blood test. If the laboratory is nearby, and if no undue delay or loss of efficiency in caring for the patient is involved, then even important blood test results should be obtained in person, not by phone.

The practicing physician should make every possible effort to secure a telephone answering service. The "service" should be instructed to call the physician only when an emergency or possible emergency exists. In addition, the practicing physician should have a separate, unlisted phone whose number he provides only to his patients classified as seriously ill, such as obstetrical patients, post-operative patients, uncontrolled diabetics, cardiacs, suicidal patients under psychiatric care, or patients suffering from similar disorders. These patients should be instructed *not* to call on this number for nonemergency needs such as scheduling of appointments. Rather, the patient should use judicious judgment and call when his physical or mental condition is such as to warrant an immediate trip to the doctor's office.

Another alternative open to the practicing physician is to hire a non-Jewish attendant to receive and make phone calls. (Also to serve as chauffeur, secretary, valet, etc.) In Israel, or where an answering service cannot be procured and where a non-Jewish attendant is not available, the following rule applies: If there are no other physicians in the area to handle the emergency needs, then the sole doctor must answer *all* phone messages because the caller may require assistance to preserve life.

The use of automatic phone recording and answering machines offers a special advantage. Since many of these instruments have a monitoring switch enabling the physician to hear the message being recorded, he can quickly decide if the caller is indeed in need of his services on the Sabbath and pick up the phone if indeed it is a case of *pikuach nefesh*.

Subject: *Use of "beepers" on the Sabbath.*

Question: May a doctor who is on call for emergencies carry a beeper to the synagogue? Is it preferable for the doctor to stay home and not attend the synagogue?

Answer and Comment: The routine carrying of a beeper on the Sabbath should be avoided unless there is an eruv in the community. The beeper can be incorporated as part of a belt—by cementing two hooks on either side of the beeper and clipping the belt onto this "buckle." It is best to have an extra beeper to leave in the synagogue to obviate the need to carry one on the Sabbath. However, if such preparations were not made, the beeper may be hooked on the belt and carried under the license that it is now part of the normal garb of a physician, analogous to the sword of a soldier (personal communication—Rav M. Feinstein).

If the doctor is "beeped" either in the synagogue or at home for an emergency, he should take a taxi to the hospital or the patient's home rather than drive his own car. However, if an undue delay is expected in securing a taxi, the physician may drive his own car.

Subject: *Turning lights on and off on the Sabbath.*

Question: Is the physician allowed to turn a light switch on, or increase the light in a patient's room in order to perform a diagnostic or therapeutic procedure? Can this be done for the patient's comfort only? Does the patient have to spontaneously make the request? May one turn off the lights afterwards?

Answer: Turning on a light is condoned on the Sabbath for a critically ill patient (*pikuach nefesh*).

Comment: Turning on a light switch or increasing the amount of light on the Sabbath is treated as an activity governed by biblical law (*d'oraitha*). Consequently, such an act can be condoned only in the case of a critically ill patient in the category of *pikuach nefesh* (danger to life). Under such conditions, the physician is obligated to provide himself with sufficient illumination to perform his diagnostic or therapeutic services in the most efficient and competent manner possible. If a non-Jew is available to turn on the room lights, he should be asked to do so.

If a patient is classified as critically ill, then even those activities associated with providing him with increased comfort are also permitted. Sabbath law is suspended for such activities, as well as for those directly associated with the care of the patient, including both diagnostic and therapeutic procedures. A sleep-disturbing lamp may be turned off to give the critically ill patient much-needed rest. If no direct benefit to the patient would result, then turning a light off on the Sabbath would be prohibited.

Subject: *Use of electric or battery-operated instruments on the Sabbath.*

Question: Is the physician permitted to turn on, operate, and use an instrument that is battery-operated or requires electric current? Can the physician turn off the instrument after he has performed the diagnostic or therapeutic procedure for which it was intended?

Answer: All instruments needed for the proper care of a critically ill patient may be used on the Sabbath.

Comment: Turning on an electrically-operated or battery-operated instrument (light- or heat-producing instruments) on the Sabbath is an act governed by biblical law, and is thus condoned only for the proper care and treatment of a critically ill patient (classified as *pikuach nefesh*). For such a patient, the physician is obligated to perform his diagnostic and therapeutic services in the most efficient manner possible, and with adequate illumination and instrumentation. If a non-Jew is available to activate such instruments, he should be asked to do so.

Instruments included in the above ruling include the following, among others:

a) ophthalmoscope-otoscope (battery-operated)
b) electrocardiograph machine (electrically-operated)
c) pacemaker-defibrillator (electrically-operated)
d) respirators (many types)
e) gastroscope-proctoscope (electrically-operated)
f) flashlight (battery-operated)

There is no basis for differentiating between battery-operated or line-operated instruments. The instruments may not be turned off on the Sabbath except by involving non-Jewish personnel, unless it is likely that the instrument will be needed again for the same or another critically ill patient. If the actual working of the instrument requires an on-off cycling by the attending physician, naturally this is permitted. However, disconnecting the instrument solely to preserve the life of the battery or bulb cannot be condoned.

Transistorized equipment avoids the halachic problem of "fire-making" that attends vacuum tube instruments, and may be preferred for this reason. However, it does present the serious halachic problem that activating an instrument is in itself a violation of the Sabbath law. Wherever feasible, it should be turned on before the Sabbath. Many instruments may be available with a "grama" switch from the Institute of Science and Halacha in Jerusalem that minimize the problem of halachic observance.

Subject: *Incision of boils and biopsies on the Sabbath.*

Question: May a boil or abscess be incised and drained on the Sabbath? May a biopsy for diagnostic purposes be performed on the Sabbath?

Answer: Only such drainage as is necessary to relieve pain and suffering is permitted on the Sabbath.

Comment: The incising of body tissue with consequent bleeding must be viewed as possibly involving biblical prohibitions. Routine biopsies of liver, skin, kidney, lymph node, etc. for diagnostic purposes would thus not be allowed.

Puncturing a boil or abscess and expressing its contents is permitted on the Sabbath, provided this is done specifically as a temporary measure to alleviate suffering. Incision and drainage of a boil or abscess, however, would constitute permanent treatment and is therefore prohibited until after the Sabbath.

Subject: *Suturing lacerations on the Sabbath.*

Question: Is one permitted to suture lacerations on the Sabbath?

Answer: Yes, lacerations may be sutured on the Sabbath.

Comment: Because of the danger of infection or possible infection, traumatic injuries of the skin, i.e., lacerations that are of sufficient magnitude to require stitches, may be repaired by suturing on the Sabbath. Since the natural history of untreated infected wounds is such that septicemia and a potentially fatal outcome may result, lacerations are considered in the category of *pikuach nefesh* (danger to life). Although the prophylactic use of antibiotics might eradicate any infection that might develop, these considerations do not remove the laceration from the category of *pikuach nefesh*, and thus it may be sutured on the Sabbath.

All the principles outlined in the next halachic answer on using antiseptic solution, tearing tape or gauze, etc., should be adhered to wherever possible.

If the injury occurs close to the end of the Sabbath, careful consultation with a rabbi who is familiar with the practice of medicine is essential.

Subject: *Injections, intravenous infusions, and blood drawing on the Sabbath.*

Question: Is the physician allowed to draw blood from someone on the Sabbath either diagnostically or therapeutically? Can procedures involving injections be performed for diagnostic (e.g., cerebrospinal tap) or therapeutic (e.g., intramuscular medications) purposes? May an intravenous injection or infusion of blood, blood products, glucose, or other solutions be administered on the Sabbath?

Answer: All the above activities involving injections, infusions, and blood drawing on the Sabbath are permitted only for patients who are classified as critically ill (*pikuach nefesh*).

Comment: The drawing of blood for tests should be viewed as involving biblical prohibitions on the Sabbath. Therefore, it should be limited to critically ill patients. The necessity of administering intravenous blood, blood products, antibiotics, chemotherapy, glucose, or other solution usually means that the patient is classified as critically ill by halachic standards. Therefore, all activities necessary for the most efficient method of accomplishing this act must be undertaken for the benefit of the patient.

Therefore, tearing tape, opening the box containing the infusion set, tearing gauze paper containers, applying antiseptic to the area of injection before and after the injection or infusion, and the like are all permitted on Sabbath. If possible, and if no loss of time or efficiency is involved, the Sabbath violations should be minimized. If it is possible to tear tape and make other preparations before the Sabbath, this should be done. If feasible, the antiseptic swab or medication should be applied in a hemostat-held gauze pad so as to approximate the situation referred to in Jewish law as a "sponge with a handle."

Phlebotomy in a polycythemic patient in whom the danger of thrombosis from high blood viscosity is being considered may be performed on the Sabbath. Elective phlebotomies should be postponed until after the Sabbath. Donation of blood by a healthy donor may be condoned only when the blood is needed immediately for a critically ill patient. Elective blood donations must wait until after the Sabbath.

Injections or removal of various body fluids such as is done in bone marrow aspirations, cerebrospinal taps, paracenteses, and the like can be performed on the Sabbath for the critically ill patient.

Subject: *Attending lectures and conferences on the Sabbath.*

Question: Is a medical student permitted to attend lectures and conferences and be present at laboratory exercises on the Sabbath, provided that he does not ride to school, take notes, or in any other way desecrate the Sabbath? Can a house officer or practicing physician attend conferences on the Sabbath with the same assumptions?

Answer: It is permitted for medical students, house officers, and attending physicians to attend lectures and conferences on the Sabbath, provided there is no violation of the laws of Sabbath observance.

Comment: A physician is required by Jewish law to acquire the maximum skill and knowledge possible to practice the highest quality medicine. The Code of Jewish Law (*Shulchan Aruch, Yoreh Deah* 336) specifically states that "no man should occupy himself with medicine unless he is well trained and there is no one better fitted than he in the place; otherwise he is shedding blood." It is not obligatory for anyone to become a physician, but once an individual undertakes to heal the sick, then he accepts the responsibilities that are entailed by the profession.

It is the responsibility and duty of the physician to treat his patients with consummate skill and competence. Any failure to achieve this competence disqualifies the individual from continuing in his role as a physician. Therefore, within the framework of halachic permissibility, the medical student or house officer must sacrifice some of the "spirit" of the Sabbath in order to obtain the maximum training in his chosen profession. With the clear understanding that there will be no violation of Sabbath law such as taking notes, operating laboratory equipment, etc., the student should attend those lectures and conferences that will add significantly to his mastery of the art and science of medicine.

The same principle applies to the physician in practice who may attend conferences on the Sabbath to maintain or improve his level of competence in medical practice, provided no Sabbath laws are violated.

The above halachic permissibility to attend conferences on the Sabbath is valid only if the conference will substantially contribute to the improvement of the student or physician's skill and competence. If the conference is merely for pleasure or general interest, and has little to offer in terms of improvement of the physician's skills, then attendance should be discouraged in favor of preserving the Sabbath spirit and engaging in the principal Sabbath activity— the study of Torah.

The availability of tapes of the lecture often obviates the need to personally attend general conferences that review known material. Conferences on the leading edge of clinical research require personal contact with the lecturers at the conference.

Subject: *Delivering a lecture on the Sabbath.*

Question: Is a physician or dentist permitted to deliver a lecture on *Shabbat* or on *Yom Tov* at a professional meeting?

Answer: If no Sabbath laws are violated, a physician or dentist is permitted to deliver a professional presentation on the Sabbath. Participation in professional conferences is an important contribution to the ongoing education of the physician.

Comment: If a physician or dentist is invited to deliver a paper or lecture on the Sabbath, he is permitted to do so provided that he does not desecrate the Sabbath in any way. Hence, he must be within walking distance and may not ride the elevator to the lecture room. He may not use a microphone or other amplifying device, nor use audiovisual material such as slide or movie projectors, and may not write on a blackboard.

He should arrange for distribution of printed or copied material in order to avoid the need for audiovisual material and in order to reduce or eliminate the need for members of the audience to take notes or tape-record the presentation. If in spite of these precautions, someone takes notes or records the presentation, the lecturer is not guilty of transgressing the negative precept of *lifnei eever lo siten michshol* (place not a stumbling block before a blind man, Lev. 19:14).

The appearance of the physician or dentist's name on the printed program does not violate any Jewish law.

Subject: *Living near the hospital for Sabbath and Yom Tov emergencies.*

Question: Must a doctor live near a hospital if he knows he may be called to see a patient on the Sabbath or can he rely on *pikuach nefesh* to travel when he gets a call? Does the probability of his being called frequently or infrequently play a role in the halachic decision?

Answer and Comment: If a physician is only rarely called to see a patient on the Sabbath or *Yom Tov* (i.e., several times a year), then he need not necessarily live within walking distance of the hospital but should respond as needed from his home or from the synagogue.

However, if he is frequently called, then it is preferable for him to live near the hospital. So too, if his synagogue is far removed from the hospital and he is frequently called for emergencies, he should stay home and not go to the synagogue because of the frequent requirement to travel via taxi to the hospital.

The definition of frequent is once a month or more, i.e., 25% of Sabbaths. If a doctor must make rounds in the hospital every Sabbath, he is obligated to live within walking distance of the hospital.

It is always strongly recommended that a non-Jewish driver or if possible a nurse or physician's assistant be employed to assist in rendering medical care on the Sabbath.

Subject: *Traveling by car to the hospital on Sabbath and Jewish holidays.*

Question: Is a physician permitted to travel by car to the hospital on the Sabbath and Jewish holidays?

Answer and Comment: If there is a dangerously ill patient in the hospital who requests a specific physician, and if that physician is already at home, it is permissible for him to ride to the hospital in any manner needed to speedily reach the patient's bedside. However, if the physician knows of such a situation on Friday, he is obligated to remain near the hospital for the Sabbath even if he must rent a room or apartment. If there is no nearby room or apartment available, he should stay in the hospital itself even if he has no wine for *Kiddush* or appropriate Sabbath meal. The commandments of *Kiddush* and the Sabbath meal cannot set aside the prohibition of desecrating the Sabbath.

However, if there is no nearby room or place in the hospital for him to sleep, he is not obligated to remain all night without sleep, since he would not be able to properly care for his patients the next day. He is no different in that respect from a teacher who is prohibited from staying up all night, since he would not be able to teach well the next day (*Ramah, Yoreh Deah* 245); all the more so for a physician who deals with danger to life. Therefore, since it is necessary for him to go home, it is permitted for the physician to travel back to the hospital since he cannot walk that far.

The above applies, however, only if the patient specifically asks for that physician or if that physician was called to care for the patient. Then it is permissible, even if other physicians are available. However, if the patient does not care which physician comes to care for him, and if that physician was not specifically called, it is certainly prohibited for him to desecrate the Sabbath.

Since there are many physicians in hospitals and since the overwhelming majority of patients are not particular about which physician cares for them and since he is not specifically called, he is not only prohibited from traveling to the hospital (by car) on the Sabbath but also prohibited from working there on the Sabbath and Jewish holidays and should try to work on another day in lieu of the Sabbath.

The use of a non-Jewish driver for returning home is strongly urged. The key consideration for permitting his return is to remove any reluctance to going initially. Since a physician has legal, professional, and social sanctions urging him to attend to his patient, the rabbinic "heter" may not be fully applicable.

Reference: Feinstein, M. *Iggrot Moshe, Orach Chayim*, New York, 1959, Responsum 131, pp. 224–225.

Subject: *Non-Jewish physician taking call on the Sabbath for a Jewish physician's patients in a group practice arrangement.*

Question: May an orthodox Jewish physician travel to his patient's bedside if his non-Jewish partner (who frequently covers for him) is available to do so on the Sabbath? What if the patient specifically requests the services of the Jewish physician even though an equally competent colleague is available and willing to care for the patient on the Sabbath?

Answer and Comment: In a group practice, the arrangement of physicians who rely on each other all week to "cover" for each other's patients assumes that the Jewish physician's responsibility for his patients on the Sabbath can be fulfilled by his assigning his non-Jewish colleague the Sabbath visits. Therefore, if the Jewish physician has full confidence that his non-Jewish partner will provide equivalent care, the Jewish physician should not travel to the hospital on the Sabbath or otherwise desecrate the Sabbath.

If a patient who is seriously ill (classified as *choleh sheyesh bo sakana*) specifically requests the Jewish physician's services, the latter must travel to the hospital, using a non-Jewish driver, to care for his patient. Even the psychological solace of added confidence in one's physician is adequate reason for permitting the setting aside of even biblical Sabbath prohibitions. If the situation is so urgent that delay in obtaining the non-Jewish driver might result in further danger to the patient's life, the Jewish physician can even drive his own car to the hospital: The physician is also permitted to return home with the non-Jewish driver.

Subject: *Treating a non-Jew on the Sabbath.*

Question: If a Jewish physician is attending a non-Jew on the Sabbath, do all exemptions from Sabbath laws that apply to a critically ill Jewish patient apply equally to the non-Jewish patient?

Answer: A Jewish physician in attendance may treat his non-Jewish patient on the Sabbath.

Comment: The Sabbath laws, both rabbinic and biblical, are set aside when a Jewish physician is actively involved in the care of any patient, Jew or non-Jew. This rule applies, of course, only in a medical situation that Jewish law (i.e., *halachah*) classifies as *pikuach nefesh* (danger to life).

Reference: *Chatam Sofer* on *Yoreh Deah* 131 (Abstract printed in margin of *Shulchan Aruch, Orach Chayim* 329).

Subject: *Training in hospitals without Sabbath obligations.*

Question: Is a physician obligated to seek training, employment, or attending physician status at a hospital where there is a minimum or no conflict between hospital policy and Sabbath observance? Should a house officer seek training at an inferior quality hospital where he is "guaranteed" not to have to work on the Sabbath or should he seek training in a hospital where training and overall patient care is far superior, but where there may be interference with the Sabbath spirit but not with the observance of halachic restrictions? Must one compromise one's medical education in order to simplify Sabbath and *kashrut* observance?

Answer: A physician must seek association with the most reputable and prestigious hospital possible to ensure excellent training and continuing education.

Comment: Jewish law requires that the physician acquire maximum skill and competence to practice his chosen profession. Therefore, he should forego the personal comfort and convenience of training in a hospital that is sympathetic to his religious needs in favor of the hospital that will provide him with the best possible training, provided that he is certain of his fortitude in maintaining all halachic requirements, despite the less favorable environment.

If the superior training is to be acquired at the price of Sabbath desecration, even of rabbinic ordinances only, the student-physician must forego the educational advantages of the prestigious hospital. It is important to emphasize that residents in non-"shomer shabbos" programs have often found themselves under great stress from hospital administrations and mentors who are unsympathetic to their religious convictions. Open discussion with the training hospital administration must be initiated before accepting such an appointment.

Subject: *Physician's fees on the Sabbath.*

Question: May a physician charge a fee for caring for a patient on the Sabbath or *Yom Tov?*

Answer: Ordinarily, the physician may *not* charge a patient for medical care on the Sabbath.

Comment: When a physician administers life-saving aid to a patient on the Sabbath or on a festival (*Yom Tov*), he cannot charge a fee because this would constitute payment for work performed on the Sabbath.

If, however, the absence of a fee "reward" would be a deterrent to the ready availability of the physician, then such a fee can be charged. This is a most sensitive point. Surely altruism is a major motivation in the choice of a medical career. However, practical considerations make for the necessity to charge a fee for medical services rendered. If the knowledge that such a fee cannot be charged for Sabbath and *Yom Tov* consultations would increase the reluctance of the Jewish physician to disturb his Sabbath and *Yom Tov* rest and lead to the rationalization that other physicians are available to be consulted, then the fee may be charged.

Needless to say, if the physician is caring for a patient over a considerable period of time that also includes Sabbath visits, he may charge a total fee to cover all services without being considered guilty of receiving remuneration for performing work on the Sabbath.

Sources: *Shulchan Aruch, Orach Chayim* 245; 246; 330:9; 407:3.

Subject: *Use of cane, crutches, walker, or wheelchair on the Sabbath and Yom Tov.*

Question: Is it permitted to go out into a public thoroughfare (*reshut harabbim*) with a cane or crutches or a walker or a wheelchair on the Sabbath? What restrictions, if any, are there?

Answer: If locomotion is impossible without them, the above mechanical aids are permitted on the Sabbath, even on a public thoroughfare.

Comment: If a paralyzed or otherwise disabled person cannot walk without a cane or crutches or a walker or a wheelchair or their like, he is permitted to go out on the Sabbath using these mechanical aids. They are treated in *halachah* like his own legs. If, however, they are used only to steady the gait of someone who can manage to walk unaided, then it is considered as if he is carrying the mechanical aid and it is prohibited on the Sabbath.

On *Yom Tov*, carrying in public does not pose a halachic problem. However, a mechanized wheelchair requires an electrical motor to be started, an activity prohibited on the Sabbath or on *Yom Tov*. Even if a non-Jew turns on the motor, there is a real concern for misinterpretation by others who will think that a Jew started the instrument (*mar'it ayin*). Hence, the use of an electric wheelchair on the Sabbath or *Yom Tov* is prohibited. A "grama" switch chair may be available from Israel.

Source: *Shulchan Aruch, Orach Chayim* 301:15, 16, and 17.

Subject: *Wearing electronic braces on the Sabbath.*

Question: *May one wear an electronic back brace on the Sabbath?*

Answer and Comment: A patient with scoliosis is allowed to wear a special electronic back brace on the Sabbath to treat the scoliosis. Such electronic back braces are available for the nonsurgical treatment of scoliosis. Sensors detect improper posture and automatically trigger a buzzer that alerts the patient to make the appropriate postural adjustment, at which time the buzzer turns itself off automatically (i.e., electronically).

Such a device does not constitute an object that the patient is "carrying" on the Sabbath but is rather considered halachically as an item of clothing. Hence, there is no prohibition of "carrying" involved. Furthermore, since no electric lights are involved and the current used is in milliamperes, all potential halachic problems are at most only rabbinical (not biblical) in nature. Hence, for medical therapeutic purposes, it is permissible to wear an electronic device as described above even if a conscious effort is used to turn off the buzzer. The automatic turning off of the buzzer is unintentional (*shelo bemiskaven*) and therefore involves no halachic prohibition on the Sabbath.

The same halachic permissibility pertains to the wearing of the T.E.N.S. electronic nerve stimulating device used for the control of intractable pain.

Subject: *Measuring one's temperature on the Sabbath and on Jewish holidays.*

Question: Is there any prohibition against measuring body temperature on the Sabbath and Jewish holidays?

Answer and Comment: The question is whether or not measuring one's temperature with a thermometer on the Sabbath is prohibited and if it is, is it a biblical prohibition. Measuring in general is not a biblical prohibition unless one is cutting to size as in following a pattern or constructing an object (*Mishneh Toreh, Hilchot Shabbat* 11:7). All other types of measurement on the Sabbath or *Yom Tov* are only prohibited by rabbinic decree (*Mishneh Torah, Hilchot Yom Tov* 4:21–22 and *Shulchan Aruch, Orach Chayim* 323). Thus, one should estimate rather than measure the amount of barley needed to feed cattle on the Sabbath and give it to them. *Tosafot* (Shabbath 126b) explains that the rabbinic prohibition against measuring on the Sabbath is only because it resembles a commercial weekday activity.

Therefore, the measurement of body temperature with a thermometer on the Sabbath does not even involve a rabbinic prohibition and to do so for a patient—even one who is not dangerously ill—is certainly permissible. For a dangerously ill patient, even biblical prohibitions would be set aside. One is not allowed to be stringent in this matter (i.e., to prohibit it), since measuring one's temperature on the Sabbath with a thermometer does not involve any prohibition at all.

Reference: Feinstein, M. *Iggrot Moshe, Orach Chayim,* New York, 1959, Responsum 128, pp. 220–221.

Subject: *High fever and Sabbath desecration.*

Question: What degree of fever warrants desecration of the Sabbath?

Answer and Comment: The Code of Jewish Law (*Shulchan Aruch, Orach Chayim* 328:7) states that one may desecrate the Sabbath for someone with high fever (i.e., who may be seriously ill). The definition of high fever is not clear. However, it is not necessary to be sure by virtue of high fever that the patient is seriously ill because even if the patient is only potentially seriously ill, one desecrates the Sabbath on his behalf. If no thermometer is available and if a person feels that he has high fever, one desecrates the Sabbath unless one is certain that he does not have high fever.

Most people feel feverish at approximately 102°F. Therefore, for 102°F one desecrates the Sabbath and one should not be strict in this matter. If someone feels feverish even at 101°F and asks that one desecrate the Sabbath for him, one should do so because it is no worse than any external injury for which one desecrates the Sabbath if the patient so requests.

In the case of a child who cannot describe a sensation of fever, if one observes that the child is extremely uncomfortable or gives other signs of illness, even if the temperature is only 100°F or above, one desecrates the Sabbath.

If the fever is due to an illness of the lungs or any other internal organ, one desecrates the Sabbath even if there is only low grade fever. But if a person has low grade fever due to an ordinary cold, one should not desecrate the Sabbath on his behalf. The opinion of a competent physician should be sought if the general malaise is more severe than expected.

Reference: Feinstein, M. *Iggrot Moshe, Orach Chayim,* New York, 1959, Responsum 129, p. 221.

Subject: *Taking medication for minor ailment on the Sabbath.*

Question: Can a patient who is allowed to take medication on the Sabbath for a serious illness also take medication for another minor ailment for which one is ordinarily not permitted to take medication on the Sabbath?

Answer and Comment: If a patient who is allowed to take medication on the Sabbath for a serious illness also suffers from another minor ailment for which one is not allowed to take medication on the Sabbath, the patient is not permitted to take the latter medication. There is no reason to allow it. In the preparation of the latter medication, one has to be concerned about biblical prohibitions such as pounding medicines, cooking, and carrying on the Sabbath.

However, if the minor ailment does not require another medication but can be treated by increasing the dose of the medication for the serious illness, one can permit the use of such an increased dose.

Reference: Feinstein, M. *Iggrot Moshe, Orach Chayim,* Part 3, 53, New York, 1973, pp. 357–358.

Subject: *Accompanying a woman in labor to the hospital on the Sabbath.*

Question: Can the husband or mother of a pregnant woman in labor accompany her on the Sabbath in a taxi to the hospital to put her mind at ease if she is fearful of going alone?

Answer and Comment: The codes of Jewish law (*Shulchan Aruch, Orach Chayim* 330:1 and *Mishneh Torah, Hilchot Shabbath* 2:11) regard a woman in labor as dangerously ill for whom the Sabbath may be desecrated. If the woman requires a light at the time when labor pains cause her to cry out, a lamp may be lit for her even if she is blind because the mere presence of a lamp will set her mind at ease. Therefore, even if the midwife claims she has no need for light, one does not rely on her expertise but lights the lamp to aid in the delivery. Certainly if the woman in labor is afraid lest the midwife err and not know what to do even if the latter is very experienced, it is required to light the lamp to put at ease the mind of the woman in labor.

Recent medical studies have shown that women whose husbands participate in the process of labor and delivery suffer fewer medical and psychiatric complications and shorter labor than if their husbands were not present.

Therefore, if she persists in her fear even after being reassured that there is no reason for her to fear traveling by herself in a taxi, there is a potential for danger to life and therefore the husband or mother should accompany her. Even if she is not yet in very active labor (literally: crying out from labor pains), if the hospital is far from her home, her husband or mother may also accompany her because, although now there may be no danger, active labor is liable to occur en route and her fear of traveling alone at that time might endanger her life.

The added weight to the car of an additional occupant requires the use of more gasoline (*marbeh beshiurim*) and would ordinarily be prohibited even if a non-Jew were driving. However, because of the danger (or potential danger) to the woman in labor, it is permitted. For the same reason we are not concerned about the law of *techum Shabbos*.

Reference: Feinstein, M. *Iggrot Moshe, Orach Chayim,* New York, 1959, Responsum 132, p. 225.

MISCELLANEOUS

QUESTIONS

Subject: *Cosmetic surgery.*

Question: Is elective cosmetic surgery permissible in Jewish law? May one undergo face-lifting surgery or nasoplasty or the like for cosmetic reasons?

Answer: If there exists a valid psychological or medical indication, elective plastic surgery for cosmetic reasons is permissible.

Comment: Without valid psychological or medical reason, undergoing elective plastic or cosmetic surgery constitutes transgression of the following prohibitions:

1) intentionally wounding oneself
2) placing one's life in possible danger

The latter prohibition must be carefully considered if the use of general anesthesia is being contemplated. The increased risk to life may indeed make such cosmetic surgery halachically unacceptable. Consultation with a competent rabbi is recommended.

Subject: *Parenteral drugs made from non-kosher sources.*

Question: Is there any prohibition in the use of parenteral medications such as pork-insulin derived from non-kosher animals?

Answer: There is *no* prohibition whatsoever involved in the use of such parenteral drugs.

Comment: There is no prohibition against *deriving benefit* from non-kosher animals. The prohibition against *eating* non-kosher food does not apply to injectables. Hence, all types of insulin, whether derived from beef or pork or other non-kosher sources, may be used without any halachic concern. The same applies to vaccines, antitoxins, etc. made from horse serum, as well as other similar parenterals.

It is remotely possible that some pharmaceuticals originate from a meat-milk mixture, e.g., beef tongue lipase, but it is most unlikely that during its preparation the halachic condition of *derech bishul* is met. Therefore, even such preparations may be used for medical treatments.

Subject: *Contact lenses and ritual immersion (tevilah).*

Question: Do contact lenses constitute an impediment to the proper performance of *tevilah?* Are such lenses considered a barrier (*chatzitzah*) between the person and the water? Must such lenses be removed before *tevilah?*

Answer: Contact lenses are considered to be a barrier (*chatzitzah*) and must be removed prior to ritual immersion.

Comment: Contact lenses are considered a barrier or separation between the water and the person performing ritual immersion. They must, therefore, be removed prior to *tevilah.* The reason for this ruling is that contact lenses are removed at prescribed intervals such as when going to bed, prior to swimming, and other such times and are, therefore, classified in the category of *makpid* (objects about which the owner cares, or is concerned to remove). It therefore follows that if contact lenses were inadvertently worn during ritual immersion (*tevilah*), competent rabbinic authority should be consulted concerning the validity of such an immersion.

Subject: *Patients who refuse blood transfusions.*

Question: If a patient appears to be dying following a massive hemorrhage or during surgery, may one administer blood or blood products to the patient if he specifically, and in writing, prohibited their use? Is one allowed to perform major surgery on a J. Witness who refuses to accept blood transfusions even at the possible cost of his life?

Answer: A Jewish physician must do all he can to save the life of Jew and non-Jew. Therefore, the physician must give blood or blood products as a life-saving procedure, even against the wishes of the patient.

Comment: The medical licensure to the physician derived from three biblical commandments (Exod. 21:19, Lev. 19:16, Deut. 22:2) requires him to exercise his best efforts. Otherwise, there might result an act of bodily injury bordering on murder. If the written refusal to accept blood transfusions is even a psychological debit to the physician or surgeon, then he should refuse to accept the case and refer the patient to another physician.

If no other physician is available, or if the Jewish physician accepts such a patient, then the wishes of the patient must become secondary to the command of God. If non-Jews are prohibited from taking even an unborn life, surely they are prohibited from taking their own life. For a patient bleeding to death, blood must be administered even in the face of written refusal of the patient.

The physician should assure his patient in advance, however, that he will respect the patient's wishes and avoid the use of blood transfusion, if at all possible, by using blood substitutes. However, if blood or blood products are deemed to be essential to the survival of the patient, then they must be administered. If the physician thereby exposes himself to legal prosecution in violating the instructions of his patient, careful consultation with competent halachic and legal authorities is essential.

Subject: *"Visiting"* the sick by telephone.

Question: Can a person fulfill the commandment of visiting the sick by speaking to the patient on the telephone?

Answer and Response: The commandment of visiting the sick in Judaism is more than just paying a social call but includes helping the patient and providing for his physical and emotional needs (see *Tur* and *Bet Yosef* on *Yoreh Deah* 335 in the name of *Ramban*). One cannot provide for these needs over the telephone. Nevertheless, if someone is unable to visit the patient at the bedside, that person partially discharges his obligation of visiting the sick because he at least performs one of the acts, i.e., comforting the patient.

One is obligated to visit in person even a patient who finds it difficult to speak because one can inquire of the patient or those attending him if there is anything that the visitor can do on behalf of the patient. Just the presence of the visitor in the room might provide comfort to the patient, such being unachievable by telephone. The visitor may also be stimulated to pray more intensely for the patient after a personal visit (Nedarim 39b–40a). Perhaps prayers are more readily answered in the patient's room because the *shechinah* (Divine Presence) is said to rest at the head of the patient's bed.

Although it is preferable to visit the patient in person, if the visitor is unable to do so or if the patient is unable to receive visitors, one is at least obligated to fulfill the obligation of *bikur cholim* as best as one can, including a telephone call.

A person cannot delegate his obligation of visiting the sick to another person, since the latter is also obliged to fulfill the commandment of *bikur cholim*. Nor should one delegate the recitation of prayers for the patient to others because all are so obligated and the more people that pray, the more likely it is that God will hear them.

Reference: Feinstein, M. *Iggrot Moshe, Yoreh Deah*, Responsum 223, New York, 1959, pp. 450–451.

Subject: *Divulging a disability to a prospective spouse.*

Question: Must a disabled person or health professional divulge health problems and issues relating to the disability to a prospective spouse? Is the discovery of the disability or health problem after marriage grounds for divorce?

Answer and Comment: Any disability that may impact negatively on the individual's functioning as spouse or parent must be revealed. Such disclosures include impairment of sexual functioning, household management, or care of children. However, the "openness" on which strong marriage bonds depend and the mutual trust and confidence that must exist between husband and wife would be seriously impaired by a failure of full disclosure of *all* matters of interpersonal concern.

Secular professional ethics may inhibit a health practitioner from sharing information about his patient's disabilities. Torah law likewise prohibits violation of confidences. However, if an intended spouse or family, concerned for the welfare of this individual, asks for information about the health status of the individual being considered for marriage, it is required to provide information limited to the areas referred to above.

Health problems that arise after marriage do not constitute grounds for divorce. However, a preexisting condition of a serious nature may indeed be *moral* and sometimes legal grounds for divorce if so evaluated by competent orthodox rabbis.

Subject: *Guide dog in the synagogue.*

Question: May a guide dog accompany its master into the synagogue?

Answer and Comment: Synagogues must not be treated disrespectfully. Ordinarily the Talmud (Megillah 28a, b) states that it is not right to eat or to drink in them. However, Raba said that the Rabbis and their disciples are permitted, since the synagogue is the "Rabbis' house." In the Jerusalem Talmud, R. Eymi invited poor travelers together with their donkeys and other belongings into the synagogue as his guests to eat and drink and rest. His opinion was that even one who is less learned than a rabbi can also consider a synagogue his house. Even bringing one's donkey or other items into the synagogue is not considered any more disrespectful than eating, drinking, or sleeping there. This ruling is found in the Codes of Jewish Law (Shulchan Aruch, Orach Chayim 151:1–14, Mishneh Berurah 151: 1–12 and others).

For urgent need (i.e., for poor people who have no home or food) it is certainly permissible to eat and drink in a synagogue. Today, even without such need, Jews have become accustomed to celebrate with food and drink the calling to the Torah of a groom on the Sabbath prior to his wedding or of a Bar Mitzvah boy. Since such customs are widely accepted throughout the Jewish world, they do not have any implication of disrespect and therefore have established legal precedent for such behavior.

There is no prohibition at all for a blind person to be accompanied by his guide dog into the synagogue. Were we to forbid it, that person would never be able to pray with a congregation, or hear the Torah or *Megillah* reading or their like. It is preferable, however, that he sit with his dog near the door so as not to disturb those fearful of animals.

When bringing an animal such as the guide dog into the synagogue is done specifically to enable its master to fulfill the commandment of public praying, there is no disrespect involved at all.

Reference: Feinstein, M. *Iggrot Moshe, Orach Chayim,* New York, 1959, Responsum 45 pp. 104–105.

Subject: *Putting on tefilin on a paralyzed arm.*

Question: Can a man whose left arm is atrophied or paralyzed don phylacteries *(tefilin)* on that arm?

Answer and Comment: It is clear that a paralyzed arm bleeds when pierced just like a healthy arm. A paralyzed arm is also not physically comparable to a "dried up" arm. The former represents an illness where the patient has no sensation in and cannot move his arm. Usually the cause for the paralysis does not lie in the arm itself but in the brain. Thus, a paralyzed arm cannot be considered missing and, therefore, one is obligated to don phylacteries thereon just as on a normal left arm. Therefore, if the left arm is paralyzed one is certainly obligated to don phylacteries thereon.

Reference: Feinstein, M. *Iggrot Moshe, Orach Chayim,* New York, 1959, Responsum 8 pp. 19–20.

Subject: *Prayers by a patient with an indwelling catheter.*

Question: May a patient with an indwelling urinary catheter recite prayers?

Answer and Comment: One should not pray or recite blessings while a stream of urine is flowing, either because of the biblical admonition *that He shall see no nakedness of anything* (Deut. 23:15), i.e., anything that one would be ashamed of, or because a stream of urine may be compared to feces and is rabbinically considered repulsive (Berachot 22b).

There is a difference of opinion as to whether a man should interrupt his prayers or even move four cubits if he is standing and reciting the *Tefilah* and he is incontinent (literally: water drips over his knees). According to *Rashba* but not *Rashi* and others, if his knees were covered by his clothes, he does not have to interrupt the recitation of *Tefilah* nor move four cubits before resuming the recitation of *Tefilah*.

Therefore, with regard to a patient with an indwelling catheter through which the urine flows into a collecting vessel, the rule of the "stream of urine" certainly does not apply. Since the urine is enclosed in the catheter, there is no embarrassment, especially since the urine flows into a closed container, i.e., the collection bag. It is preferable for the collection bag to be covered, but if that is not possible, it is permissible for the patient to recite his prayers even if it is not covered. However, the catheter itself should be covered.

Reference: Feinstein, M. *Iggrot Moshe, Orach Chayim,* New York, 1959, Responsum 27 pp. 71–72.

Subject: *Expert non–Torah observant physician.*

Question: What principles govern whether to consult a Torah observant physician or an expert physician who does not observe the precepts of the Torah?

Answer and Comment: If the choice is between two physicians, one who observes the precepts of the Torah but is not a specialist and another who is a specialist but is not Torah-observant and is in fact an atheist (*kofer*), who should the patient consult?

This question requires no lengthy reply. The Torah permits one to seek healing from physicians. According to Maimonides and others, it is obligatory to do so. Therefore, one should go to the most expert physician, even if he is an atheist.

We should not wonder how or why God sends healing through the hands of an atheist because in case of illness, we are divinely commanded not to rely on a miracle as long as we can be healed with a remedy that God created. This (atheist or irreligious) physician is familiar with the illness and knows best which remedies to apply to cure it.

In regard to a possible error by the physician, one should pray to God that the physician not err and that his healing should be successful. The Talmud states (Abodah Zarah 28a) that Jews in those days sought healing from pagan and apostate physicians without fear that the latter might harm them.

But if the physician is one who suborns heresy (*mesis umayde'ach*), it is forbidden to go to him to seek healing even if there is no other physician. However, the overwhelming majority of physicians, whether Gentile or irreligious Jews, perform their healing tasks appropriately and have nothing to do with religious heresy.

Reference: Feinstein, M. in *Sefer Halachah Urefuah* (Halachah & Medicine), Ed. M. Hershler, Jerusalem-Chicago, Regensberg Institute, 1980, p. 130.

LISTING OF MEDICAL RESPONSA

OF RAV MOSHE FEINSTEIN

IN HIS *IGGROT MOSHE*

BIBLIOGRAPHY

OF MEDICAL

HALACHIC BOOKS IN ENGLISH

1. Jakobovits, J. *Jewish Medical Ethics*. New York: Bloch, 1975; 439 pp.
2. Feldman, D. M. *Marital Relations, Birth Control and Abortion in Jewish Law*. New York: Schocken, 1975; 322 pp.
3. Rosner, F. *Modern Medicine and Jewish Law*. New York: Bloch for Yeshiva University Press, 1972; 216 pp.
4. Bleich, J. D. *Contemporary Halakhic Problems*. New York: Ktav and Yeshiva University Press, 1977; 403 pp.; Vol. 2, 1983, 423 pp.
5. Landman, L. (editor) *Judaism and Drugs*. New York: Federation of Jewish Philanthropies, 1973; 269 pp.
6. Rosner, F. *Medicine in the Bible and the Talmud*. New York: Ktav and Yeshiva University Press, 1977; 247 pp.
7. Hankoff, L. D. (editor) *Jewish Ethno-Psychiatry*. New York: Federation of Jewish Philanthropies, 1977; 80 pp.
8. Rosner, F., and Bleich, J. D. *Jewish Bioethics: A Book of Essays*. New York: Hebrew Publishing Co., 1979; 424 pp.
9. Tendler, M. D. *Pardes Rimonim (a marriage manual for the Jewish family)*. New York: Judaica Press, 1977; 93 pp. 2nd edit. 1988.
10. Preuss, J. *Biblical and Talmudical Medicine*, transl. F. Rosner. New York: Hebrew Publishing Co., 1978; 688 pp.
11. Abraham, A. S. *Medical Halachah for Everyone*. Jerusalem: Feldheim, 1980; 232 pp.
12. Spero, M. H. *Judaism and Psychology: Halakhic Perspectives*. New York: Ktav and Yeshiva University press, 1980; 275 pp.
13. Bleich, J. D. *Judaism and Healing: Halakhic Perspectives*. New York: Ktav, 1981; 199 pp.
14. Feldman, D. M., and Rosner, F. *Compendium on Medical Ethics*. New York: Federation of Jewish Philanthropies, Sixth Edition, 1984; 149 pp.
15. Rosner, F. *Modern Medicine and Jewish Ethics*. New York: Ktav and Yeshiva University Press, 1986; 405 pp.
16. Sokol, B. *Halakha and Medicine. A Physician's Manual. Hilchot Shabbat*. Jerusalem: Regensberg Institute, 1986; 307 pp.
17. Feldman, D. M. *Health and Medicine in the Jewish Tradition*. New York: Crossroad, 1986; 114 pp.
18. Meier, L. *Jewish Values in Bioethics*. New York: Human Sciences Press, 1986; 195 pp.

GLOSSARY OF

HEBREW AND ARAMAIC

TERMS AND PHRASES

Aliyah: going to settle in Israel.

Amirah le'akum: telling a non-Jew (to perform an act prohibited to a Jew on the Sabbath).

Basar, gidim, ve'atzamot: flesh, sinews and bones (if present in an excised organ or limb, dictate burial of that organ).

Bemakom tzar lo gozru bo rabbanan: when there is pain (or discomfort) the rabbis did not enact prohibitions.

Bikur cholim: visiting the sick.

Bohul al gufoh: concern for one's body.

Brit or Brit Milah: ritual circumcision.

Chametz: leavened products containing wheat, barley, rye or oats.

Chatzitzah: a foreign body such as adhesive tape or cosmetics that must be removed before ritual immersion known as *tevilah.*

Chavalah: wound or wounding.

Chayey sha'ah: short term survival of a dying patient.

Chesron eyver: loss of function of an organ or limb.

Choleh: sick person.

Choleh She'ayn bo sakanah: patient in whom there is no danger to life.

Choleh She'ayn bo sakanah im tzar gadol: patient in whom there is no danger to life but who is suffering with great pain and discomfort.

Choleh Sheyesh bo sakanah: patient who is ill with a potentially fatal disease.

Chol Hamo'ed: intermediate days of the holidays of Passover and Tabernacles.

Davar She'ayn miskaven: an unintential act.

Davening: praying (Yiddish).

Dechuya: temporary suspension (of Sabbath laws).

Derech bishul: in the manner of cooking.

D'oraitha: biblical (law).

Ducheka desakina: literally: pressure of a knife.

Eruv: a legal method to enable people to carry on the Sabbath in a public thoroughfare.

Eyvorim: limbs or organs (of the body).

Fleishig: meat foods or utensils (Yiddish).

Frum: orthodox (Yiddish).

Gadol Hador: rabbinic leader of the generation.

HaGaon: the extraordinary biblical scholar.

Hakoras tov: showing one's gratitude for favors or kindnesses.

Halachah: Jewish law.

Halachic: pertaining to Jewish law.

Hatofat dam: blood flow during ritual circumcision.

Hefsed mamom: monetary loss.

Heter: permissible ruling.

Hutra: abrogation (of Sabbath laws).

Issurei d'rabbanan: rabbinic prohibitions.

Kashrut: permissibility (possessive form of *Kosher*).

Kiddush: sanctification (of the Sabbath with a cup of wine).

Kofer: (plural: *kofrim*): agnostic(s) or atheist(s).

Kohen: (plural: *kohanim*): priest(s).

Kol tzorchei choleh: all the needs of the patient.

Lefanenu: at hand, (literally: before us).

Lifney eever lo siten michshol: place not a stumbling block before a blind
   man (Lev. 19:14).

Lishah: kneading (a forbidden task on the Sabbath).

Ma'aseh Uman: act of an expert.

Maga: touching.

Makah shel chalal: internal sore or wound.

Makpid: punctilious, concerned, strict.

Mapis mursa: incision of an abscess.

Marbeh beshiurin: increasing the amount.

Marit ayin: outward appearance (literally: the eye sees).

Massa: carrying.

Mechatech basar be'alma: cutting off loose flesh.

Megillah: biblical book of Esther (literally: scroll).

Memachek: smoothing or waxing.

Mesis umayde'ach: one who leads Jews astray (from Judaism).

Metaken manah: improving or forming a utensil.

Metzitzah: sucking the wound following circumcision.

Meychush be'alma: minor discomfort.

Mikvah: ritualarium for ritual immersion.

Milchig: dairy foods or utensils (Yiddish).

Minim: aggressively irreligious people.

Mishkav zachor: homosexuality.

Mitzvah: commandment or meritorious act.

Mohel: (plural *mohalim*): ritual circumciser(s).

Mutal lemishkav: as if confined to bed.

Nefel: non-viable fetus or neonate.

Niddah: ritual uncleanliness during menses and for seven days thereafter.

Nivul hamet: desecration of the dead.

Pesik reysho: unavoidable result of an act (literally: cut off the head).

Pikuach nefesh: danger to life.

Psak: rabbinic ruling.

Rav: rabbi.

Reshut harabbim: public thoroughfare.

Sapheck: doubt.

Shabbat or *Shabbos:* the Sabbath.

Shabbos goy: non-Jew who performs acts on the Sabbath for a Jew (or Jews).

Shechinah: Divine Presence.

She'elah-teshuvah (plural: *She'elot-teshuvot*): question(s) and answer(s).

Shelo bemiskaven: without intent.

Shenayim she'osu: two people performing a single act.

Shinuy: performing an act (on the Sabbath) in an unusual manner.

Shofar: ram's horn.

Shul: synagogue.

Sirus: castration.

Techum Shabbos: area within a city within which it is permitted to walk on the Sabbath.

Tefilah: prayer.

Tefilin: phylacteries worn during daily morning prayer service.

Tevilah: ritual immersion.

Tumat ohel: ritual defilement by being present in the same room as a corpse.

Yad Soledet bo: an object sufficiently hot that the hand recoils when it touches it.

Yarok beyoter: excessively jaundiced.

Yoledet: parturient woman.

Yom Tov: Jewish holiday.

Zt'l: of blessed and sainted memory.

About the Authors

Dr. Fred Rosner is Director of the Department of Medicine of the Mount Sinai Services at the Queens Hospital Center and Professor of Medicine at New York's Mount Sinai School of Medicine. Dr. Rosner, an internationally known authority on medical ethics, has lectured widely on Jewish medical ethics. He is the author of six widely acclaimed books on Jewish medical ethics, including *Modern Medicine and Jewish Ethics* and *Medicine and Jewish Law*. These books are up-to-date examinations of the Jewish view on many important bioethical issues in medical practice. Dr. Rosner is also a noted Maimonidean scholar and has translated and published in English most of Maimonides' medical writings.

Dr. Moshe D. Tendler serves in a dual capacity as Professor of Biology at Yeshiva University in New York City and as a *rosh yeshiva* (Professor of Talmud) at the University-affiliated Rabbi Isaac Elchanan Theological Seminary (RIETS). Dr. Tendler also serves as rabbi of the Community Synagogue in Monsey, New York. He and his wife, Sifra, are the parents of eight children.